HEALTHY MOM…
…SICK MOM

By:

Chronic Mom

Cover Photo By: Chronic Mom

DEDICATION

I dedicate this book to all those who are suffering from any kind of autoimmune disease, chronic illness, chronic pain, and motherhood. You have a beautiful soul, so keep up the fight.

I also dedicate this book to my husband and sons. You are my rock and every day I will continue to fight and show you that nothing can take me down.

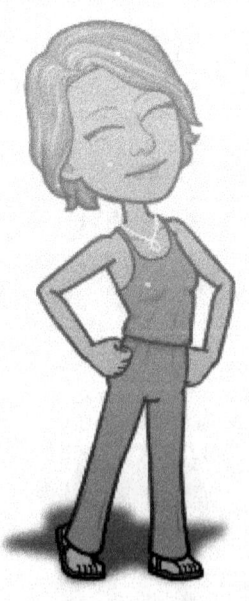

CONTENTS

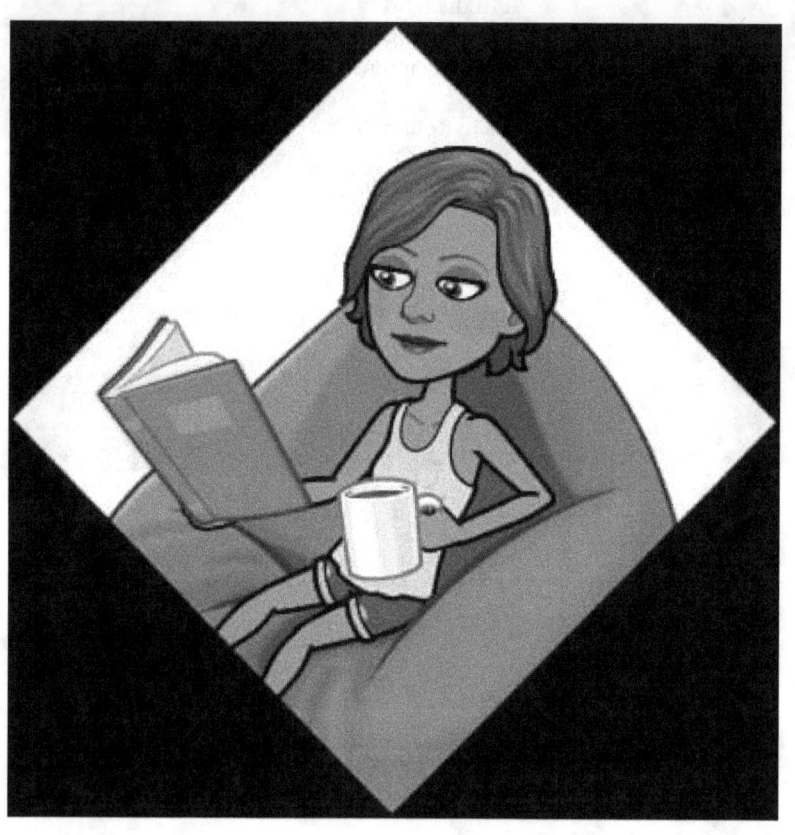

OTHER BOOKS BY CHRONIC MOM

Fighting Addisons Disease and Fibromyalgia:
My 50 day journey on a whole food plant based diet.

INTRODUCTION

No one ever expects to get sick. We just live our lives thinking (hoping) that nothing bad will happen to us. Sure, we think about car accidents, breaking a limb, or things of that nature, but never can we plan for something like an autoimmune diseases, cancers, or heart attacks.

When I found out that I had Addison's Disease, my first thought was, "at least it's not cancer." A close friend said to me, "You can't look at it that way. Cancer is different. People can get treatment and beat cancer; Addison's Disease is a life sentence. There is no cure and your body could shut down because of stress and you could slip into a coma or die.... Just from stress. So, don't take what you have lightly." She was right, and living with this disease has been a real eye opener for me.

I didn't know anything about Addison's Disease. I just knew that I had to take some pills and see my Endocrinologist every 3-4 months to make sure all my levels were good. The Dr. told me "try not to get sick, don't get stressed, and don't get into any accidents." All things that I have no control over. He never really gave me an explanation as to why I am not supposed to do those things, and I didn't ask. I was not taking this disease seriously, even though I could feel it affecting me.

About 2 years later I was diagnosed with Fibromyalgia. Really? Another autoimmune? They will just keep piling on; and through the years, I will just get worse. This is the reality that I have to live in. This is my new life. The life that I am still supposed to try and function in. The life I have to raise 3 boys in.

I always try to think that "I got this," and that the disease does not have me, I am my own person and I control it. But in reality, it has me. I am always trying to hide the fact that I can't fight anymore. This is where I feel like I should be winning an Oscar for my performance. It's not easy to fake it every day. It's not easy to walk around like you are not feeling the pain that tortures you. It's not easy hanging out with friends and acting like you are having a good time, when all you want to do is scream "AAAHHHHHHH, MAKE IT STOP!!" But we do, every…single…fucking…day.

I got to be a healthy mom, just not for as long as I wanted to. Now, I am a sick mom, and my journey has changed.

FIRST TIME MOM

When I was growing up, I babysat for a couple families in the town I grew up in. I was never a "baby person" and I didn't really like little kids, but every teenager needs to earn money, so this is what I did until I was old enough to work at the local restaurant.

I hated babysitting and there were these 2 boys I watched that were HORRIBLE. Think Dennis the menace times 2. Not only did I watch them, we also had my best friend's nieces living with us (I lived with my best friend and her family from 8th grade until graduation). Those two girls were a handful as well. Kids were just not something I was interested in. I wasn't even sure if I wanted to have kids. I wanted to travel and be able to have freedom and no responsibilities.

That all changed really quickly when I graduated from high school and met my first husband at the end of June 1999 (just a couple weeks after I graduated). We started dating in July. It was new, he was from Western Washington, he was athletic and handsome, and gave me all the feels. We both wanted to wait until we were married to have sex, but that didn't happen. I will say that we were engaged, we just didn't make it to the wedding night. Our wedding was set for October 24, 1999. He was leaving for boot camp and we wanted to get married before he left. We started having sex soon after he proposed in August. A week before the wedding, I found out I was pregnant.

This really freaked me out. I was told that I would have a hard time getting pregnant. My senior year I had a huge cyst on my ovary that had to be removed. The Dr. said that there was some damage left and that I would have a harder time getting pregnant......LIAR!!!! I still was not sure I wanted to have kids, and now, it was too late. I had a tiny human growing inside of me and my soon to be husband would be leaving for boot camp for 12 weeks. I knew nothing about pregnancy and how it would affect me. I had a few books that I looked through, but never read. None of my friends had ever gone through this. We were all only 18-19 years old. I was not ready to be a mom. I didn't even have my shit figured out yet.

I was sick the whole pregnancy. It was a nightmare. I hated every minute of it. I couldn't eat, every smell either made me sick or made me want to eat (and eating made me sick), I couldn't sleep because I was so uncomfortable, I cried all the time (and I am not a crier), and I didn't have my husband around to help me through this.

He finally got done with boot camp in February and came home for 2 weeks and then had to leave again for training. I felt so alone in this pregnancy (that I wasn't enjoying). I thought I was going to be a horrible mom. I was just miserable.

We were given permission to get a house off base since the baby was due at the end of May (we couldn't live in base housing because he was only there for training). I moved down to 29 Palms California with him in the beginning of April. We knew we still had over a month before our son was born. It was so hot. I sat in our tiny studio apartment, that only had a swamp cooler, in my underwear and bra, while he was at training.

Contractions started happening often and I had no clue what was going on. I ignored it, thinking it was just stomach pains. Finally, I went in and they checked me. I was already dilated to 2 and it was only April 23rd. I still had a month to go. I wasn't ready to have a baby early. The contractions just started getting worse and I rested as much as I could. I was so scared of what would happen.

At 6am on April 27th, I woke up in a lot of pain. I had my husband take me to the hospital. They checked me, and I was still only dilated to 2, but the nurse looked very confused. She smiled and said, "let me get the Dr. and see what she says." Not knowing anything about giving birth, I didn't think anything of it, yet I had a weird feeling about the nurse's reaction. My husband had to go into school at 7am, so when he left, I was there alone. We didn't have any family or friends around.

The Dr. didn't come in until about 8:30am. She checked me and said, "Oh. Well, you are only dilated to 2, but I can feel his head. He is coming. I am not sure what to do."

My eyes felt like they burst out of my head. I couldn't believe what she just said. She didn't know what to do? Was she expecting me, a 19-year-old, first time mom, with no medical background, to know what to do? I was internally freaking out.

Then she said, "I'll be right back."

I wanted to scream and cry. I wanted to get up and walk out of there. I was scared out of my mind. My husband wasn't there to comfort me. I couldn't call anyone. It was just me.

She finally came back in about 45 mins later and said they were going to give me Pitocin to help me dilate. Finally, we had a plan and I felt a little better, but I was still worried about his poor little head just sitting there. I wanted to ask if he would be able to breath, or if there was going to be some complication if he sat there too long. I didn't understand the whole layout of where he was, but the vagina doesn't seem to be the best place for a baby to just be hanging out.

Once the Pitocin kicked in (around 11am), I was in a whole lot of pain. They wanted to wait til I was at 4 cm before they broke my water, and they said that would help speed things along too. That was an extremely painful experience. It felt like she was trying to stab and kill me through my vagina. I was also worried about my baby being poked and his head being damaged by that crochet needle looking thing.

Things were not moving fast. My husband came up from school for his lunch and was able to stay with me the rest of the time. I was begging for an epidural at this point. The pain was way too much for my body to handle and I just wanted it to stop. When the anesthesiologist was doing the epidural, my husband was the one I was holding onto. All of a sudden, I hear the nurse ask, "Are you ok?" When I started to look up to answer her, she had moved pretty quickly over to my husband and had him by the arm. He almost passed out. He was flushed and completely white (even whiter than he was). I can't believe that he was going to pass out, just from watching me get an epidural. Really? I am here, in pain, having a gigantic needle shoved in my back, and he is going to pass out? Good thing us ladies have the babies.

Once they were done and got the medicine in, she waited about 2 min and then, she started scratching my leg and asking if I could feel anything. I said yes, since I could feel her scratching me with her nail. She gave me more medicine and waited about 2 min again and repeated scratching my leg. I could still feel it. So, she put in another dose and said, "Might take a bit more since you are so tall." I of course had no clue what that meant, but I was counting on her to know what she was doing. This time she waited about 5 min. Finally, I felt the meds kicking in and I was pretty happy that I couldn't feel the contractions any more. I also couldn't feel my legs. It was like they weighed 500lbs (come to find out later that she didn't wait long enough for the meds to kick in and she gave me WAY too much because of it).

The Dr. came in and checked on me a few times to see if I was dilating, and I was, but it was such a slow process, so she kicked up the Pitocin. I was so happy that I was not feeling it anymore and I was able to get a little bit of rest.

Finally, at about 3am I was ready to push. 10 cm had finally come. Thanks to the overdose on the epidural, I was not able to push like I was supposed to. They kept telling me to push harder and I tried, but I just couldn't. My husband kept trying to look at the progress of the birth, and I was trying to keep him by my head. He didn't need to be seeing my vagina all stretched out and disgusting looking.

The Dr. used this vacuum thing to try and help and she also used the forceps. He was just not coming. She ended up having to give me an episiotomy.

At 4:02am I had a beautiful 6 lb. 1 oz. baby boy. I was so exhausted. When he slid out, he was not crying. They spanked him and nothing. They wiped him up really quick and had 2 nurses with the nose sucker thing working on him, trying to get him to cry. They decided to wheel him out and my husband went with him. The Dr. told me everything would be ok, but I was so scared. I didn't know what to expect and I just wanted my baby to be ok.

The Dr. said "ok, I need you to push again."

I gave her the most confused look. "Is there another baby in there?" I asked. I had no clue why I had to push again. She laughed and said "Nope, you just need to push out the placenta."

Oh, thank God. Because there was no way I could push out another baby.

After I pushed out the placenta she asked me if I wanted to see it and she held it up, like it was a baby. Why they hell would I want to see the placenta? It was so nasty looking.

They got everything cleaned up and I sat there, wondering, what was happening to my son. Was he ok? Was he breathing? Was there something wrong because he wasn't crying?

About an hour later, my husband and a nurse came in with my baby boy. He was so tiny. I didn't realize how small he would be. I was wondering where all of him had gone. I unwrapped him to make sure he was all there, because a baby shouldn't be that small. He was beautiful. He had all his parts and was perfect. They said he was just tired from trying to get out and he was a healthy little boy.

Once I saw him, my heart felt like it was going to explode. I never wanted to let him go. He was my everything. I fell in love for the first time. I never wanted this perfect little angel to leave my sight again.

The next day he had his circumcision and he apparently slept through that. Childbirth was hard on him. He was trying to get out for a few days and that just tuckered him out. At his 3-day check-up, they noticed that he was really jaundice. They admitted us back into the hospital and we were there for 3 days. He had to stay under the Bilirubin lights. I wasn't allowed to hold him unless I was feeding or changing him. I felt horrible. I couldn't even hold my own baby. He just had to lay there, unwrapped, not being held.

When we took him home, they sent us with a Bilirubin light machine that he had to lay on. I was able to keep that light on him and hold him at the same time. I just couldn't get enough of him. I couldn't stop looking at him, I didn't want to put him down. I never knew being a mom would feel like this. He was now my whole world and I would die before I let anything, or anyone hurt him.

MOM: ROUND 2

I am so happy that going through labor the 2nd time was a whole lot easier than the first. I was hell bent on not doing it at a military hospital again. Once was enough for me and I wanted Drs. who knew what they were doing and not in a place where it was a "learning experience."

I wish I could say the 2nd pregnancy was easier than the first. Again, I was sick the whole time. My oldest son was there with me in the bathroom as I threw up. He would rub my back and say, "It's ok mommy." He was the sweetest little thing.

I did take up running with this pregnancy to help myself stay in better shape and to make giving birth a little easier. With my first I was not motivated to workout at all. I was sick the entire time, my husband was off at boot camp, all my friends were out partying…. No fun for this mama.

My husband was around for this one, but I am sure he wishes he wasn't. I cried over every little thing. I made him wake up at 3am to go get me sausage McMuffins (I craved those so bad). I remember one time he came back and told me they didn't open til 5am, and I cried, so he said he would go drive around til he found one that was open. My guess was that he just went and slept in the car til 5am.

I couldn't stand the site or smell of chicken, so we gave up eating that til after I had the baby. I was so mean and emotional (think of Rachel from *Friends* at the end of her pregnancy…That was me the whole time). I think he thought I was crazy.

With this pregnancy I fell in love with running and working out. It really helped my mood and got me out and about. Me and my husband were youth leaders at a church in Missouri. I didn't know this til after I had my son, but the kids were afraid of me. They thought I was so mean and they would try to avoid me (a few liked me and could stand the meanness). We did a bunch of fundraisers and one that was my favorite was the fireworks tent. It was so hot and there were so many people who would ask stupid questions. Not the best place for a pregnant woman to be working at. I was asked a few times to be nice to the customers.

I got a job at a hotel and really enjoyed working there. My manager was scared of me and tried to avoid me, because he didn't want me yelling at him. I remember having to be moved to the back office and given the job of answering phones because guests were complaining about the angry pregnant lady at the front desk (told you I was mean). My boss was trying to say it in the nicest way and ended up chickening out and having the front desk manager tell me. He was this amazing gay guy who just gave it to me straight. "You need to work back here and answer phones because, even though you are sweet and the cutest pregnant girl ever, you have attitude that the guests don't like. Although I find it amusing, they don't." I loved him so much.

I liked Missouri better than I liked California. The people were nicer, the area was beautiful, and we were able to live on base (after housing had opened up for us. We were in an apartment for a while at first). I really liked my Dr. and we had made a lot of friends within our church group. Our associate Pastor and his wife would take our oldest and make us go out on date nights. It was so hard leaving our little guy, but they told us not to come back for 3 hours. It was nice to have people who cared about us around. Our Youth Pastors wife had found out that we had been sleeping on a blow-up mattress that kept deflating, and she brought it up to the Main Pastor. They ended up buying us a bed to sleep on. They didn't want a pregnant woman, who they have come to love, sleeping on the floor like that. Such kindness and love they showed us unconditionally.

When it came time for this birth, I had a plan. I was going to do this natural. With the trauma that had happened with the epidural the first time, I didn't want to have to go through that again. My son's due date was October 23, 2002. My friend and I were only 1 day apart from our due dates and we were excited, hoping our kids would be born on the same day. My sister/best friend was due at the beginning of July, so all 3 of our kids would be really close in age. This was something that we thought would be cool when we were in middle school, and it ended up actually happening. Unfortunately, we all lived in different places, but it was still exciting that we all were having our babies so close together.

Towards the end of September, I started having contractions. They were pretty painful. I was dilated to 2 cm and the Dr. put me on bed rest. They didn't want this baby coming to early. With having my first one a month early and everything being ok with him, we weren't too worried about it. Around 3am on September 27th, I was in labor. I just can't seem to keep these babies in long enough.

We went into the hospital, hoping for a different outcome for this little guy. They asked me if I wanted an epidural and I refused, I wanted to do this all natural. After 5 hours, the contractions were so close together and I wasn't dilating, they decided to break my water to help speed things along. I was so scared to have to go through this again. Luckily, the guy who did it, was a pro. It didn't hurt nearly as much as the first time.

After 7 hours and still no dilation, they started pushing the Pitocin. This is where I lost it. The increased pain had me screaming. I wasn't sure if I was going to make it. They told me I had until 6 cm to decide if I wanted an epidural. They offered me other pain meds and I gladly took them. I still felt all the pain, but I was so drugged that my response was just a "oww. This hurts" in a very "high" state. Finally, the pain got to be too much, and I caved. I asked for an epidural. Thankfully I was only dilated to a 4 cm when they checked and gave the go ahead to the anesthesiologist. They came in to do the epidural and I was at 6 cm now. I was dilating fast, so I was happy to get the meds going.

Before the meds had fully kicked in, I told my husband that I felt like I needed to push. There was so much pressure on my vagina that I couldn't help it and it felt like my vagina was on fire. He called the nurse in and she looked, the baby was crowning. She got the Dr. in and here I was ready to push out this baby.

I was scared because the epidural had not fully kicked in and I could feel the pain still. I didn't want to feel the pain, but it was too late. He was coming and he was coming fast.

I pushed about 15 times and he was out. He was so tiny, but he had a set of lungs on him. I was so thankful to hear his little cry. I watched as they cleaned him up a bit and then they brought him to me. My heart again was so full of love. He was so beautiful. He had so much light brown and blonde hair and his little face was perfect. His eyes were such a beautiful blue. He weighed 5lbs 12oz and was born at 5:12pm. Another perfect son.

Thankfully he was as healthy as could be. No jaundice issues, he cried when he needed to, and he handled his circumcision like a normal baby would. I created another perfect angel.

MOM: FINAL ROUND

This little gem was such a surprise. I know now, that this one was supposed to be born. He found his way to me, a true gift from God. Not that I don't love my other boys, but this one was sent to teach me a lesson.

Get ready for some TMI.

I had just separated from my first husband and was "dating" this one guy. We were having fun, but he was too much of a partier for me. He drank like a fish, a true functioning alcoholic. He was one of those guys you have fun with but don't want a serious relationship with. He had a daughter who was the same age as my second son. He was a weekend dad and he really enjoyed that, because he didn't want the responsibility of having her all the time (a real winner- Red flags EVERY WHERE). This is the last guy I would have EVER wanted to have a baby with.

I was on the pill and he pulled out, just to be safe…. Nope. I was pregnant within a few months of seeing him. W…T… FUCK!!!!! I was so disappointed. At the time I had a roommate and I told her, when I found out, that I was just going to break up with him and he would never have to know. I know how messed up that was, but I didn't want to have a baby with him.

When I told him, he freaked out a little bit and then said, "You can just get an abortion." Like it was even an option for me. NOPE. NOT HAPPENING. Sorry, but I could NEVER EVER do something like that. I was no position to be having a child, and obviously he did not want one. I was barely making ends meet and I was also a weekend mom. I could barely afford to pay attention. How the hell was I supposed to take care of a baby?

I was working at a gym at the time and had made friends with this amazing couple. I had opened up to her about my fears, and she told me they had friends who were looking to adopt. She set up a meeting with them, so I could meet and talk about them possibly adopting my baby.

The baby daddy dropped me off, he didn't even want to come in and meet them, he could have cared less what happened. I met and talked with them. They were amazing. They both made a lot of money, loved to travel, had a big beautiful house. I wanted them to adopt me. When I left, I was a little sad and mad. Mad at myself for getting into this situation and sad because I didn't want this baby to ever feel that it wasn't loved. I knew that the adoptive parents would be amazing, but what if one day he came looking for me and asked why I gave him up?

A few days later I saw the friend who had set up the meeting and she told me that they didn't want to adopt my baby. She told me, "They said you talked about your older boys with so much love and they could tell you were an amazing mom. They said no one will love this baby more than you and you needs to keep it."

I was so touched, and it made me realize they were right. I loved my boys so much, they were my heart beat, my breath, my everything. This one would be the same, just a little harder to do on my own.

I told the baby daddy I was keeping the baby and he didn't have to be involved at all. He thought about it for a couple days and then the asshole said "let's get married. I want to do this the right way and give this baby a family." DA FUCK DUDE…. Back up just a bit here… My divorce was just finalized 5 days ago. And this guy, who wanted me to have an abortion and didn't even come to see about the adoptive parents, now wants to marry me. HAHAHAHAHAHA!!! No thank you.

I told him, "sure, ya, let's do that. Let's go to the courthouse and get married." Gaging what his reaction would be, because I knew he had to be joking. We talked about it and I told him that it would be best to maybe just move in together and see if we can even tolerate each other.

A couple months after I moved in with him, I called my friend and told her to come get me. I moved in with my mom and got a job. His job was transferring him to Eastern Washington, so he told me to find us a place there and we could work this out. I was not convinced, but I was also scared to do this on my own. I found us a place and the asshole moved into it and said, "We shouldn't live together, you need to find your own place."

And that ended our relationship.

This pregnancy was lonely, but I made some really good friends. I was working as the head teacher in the toddler room at a daycare, so it was pretty easy. I was not making a lot of money, but enough to keep a studio apartment and some food on the table.

When I was 26 weeks, I started having contractions really bad. My doctor wanted to put me on bed rest, but I was a single mom and I couldn't do that. My boss hired me an assistant and I was able to have her do most of the lifting and harder work, while I sat there.

At 27 weeks I went into labor. I was flown to Tacoma, because the hospital I was going to have him at in Wenatchee, wasn't equipped to handle a baby being born under 36 weeks. They were able to stop labor. My best friend/sister drove over to be with me, just in case I had the baby.

I was able to keep him in, barely, to the 36-week mark. My Dr. broke my water at 3pm and I was not dilating, so I got to have some Pitocin. I was doing a natural birth, so no epidural for me. It was so painful. All you moms who have had to have Pitocin know that it intensifies the contractions. My best friend/sister was there and one of the moms from the daycare I worked at. They were so amazing and helped me through the painful labor.

When it came time to push, my best friend/sister was so hopped up on adrenalin, she about passed out and went into the bathroom and I do believe she was throwing up but came out just in time to see my little guy slide out.

He was perfect and beautiful. My best friend/sister and the mom told me that I needed to let the dad know. Even though he was a dickface, he had the right to come see his son. I let him know and he came up to see him. I knew that I would have to do this alone, so I asked the nurse to take the baby away when I was done feeding him, so I could rest as much as possible before they sent me home the next day. Baby daddy left when they took him. The nurse came in a few hours later with the baby again and said that baby daddy stayed and watched in the window of the nursery for about an hour. I was really shocked, but I also knew what a good manipulator he was.

He saw the baby a couple times after we got home. He brought his daughter over to meet him when he was about 6 weeks old. The jerk had the nerve to ask me to have sex with him in my bathroom while his daughter sat with the baby. I KNOW RIGHT! I didn't want him to be anywhere near my son. Not long after that he asked if I would be ok with him signing over his rights because he didn't want to have to pay child support for another kid. I looked into it and unfortunately, that can't happen unless someone is adopting him. Tough luck asshole, you are stuck. I should have taken him for all of it, but I am too nice of a person and only made him pay $200 a month.

My son is an amazing kid, has a great dad (who wanted him and adopted him when he was 2), and never has to meet his biological father if he doesn't want to. He knows that he exists, but at 9 years old, he still has no desire to know him and I am fine with that. I don't talk bad about him (or really ever mention him at all) and we actually see his family still, but he is not allowed around my son. His own daughter even stopped seeing him a couple years ago.

This pregnancy was my "easiest" but definitely had the most drama to it.

I am so glad that I was able to be a healthy mom for the first 4 ½ years of his life. I was able to do all the important mom things for him as he grew in those first years when he really needed all of me. Had I been sick then, I don't think I would have made it.

He takes care of me on most days, which breaks my heart, because no 9-year-old should have to do that, but I am thankful that he can and that he still remembers when we use to do so many things together.

SCARED MOM

On Memorial Day 2018, I was shopping at Dick's Sporting Goods with all 3 of my boys. My body was already really sore from the fun we had on Saturday and all the traveling. I was looking at bikes and I called my youngest over to come look. As I was trying to pull a bike out, my son decided to "go missing," we couldn't find him. I stayed in that area, hoping he would come back, and sent my older 2 boys to look through the store.

As I stayed, I was looking around for him. There was this woman there with her 2 daughters, talking to a salesman. About 8 min had passed and all of a sudden, I hear a scream.

"MOMMY!! MOMMY!! HELP ME! MOMMY HELP ME!"

This scream was one of a very scared and crying child. My heart sunk as I realized it was my son screaming. His voice was muffled, like he was far away. I looked around and noticed the bathrooms right there. Every horrible thought crossed my mind. I didn't even think, I just ran into the men's room and yelled my son's name. I could see his shorts were dropped around his ankles and he was standing by the door of the stall, but still inside of it.

"Are you ok?!?!" I shouted; panicking.

"The light turned off. I got scared," he said. He was crying, and his voice was staggered, heavy breathing, and he was terrified.

"Ok. It's back on. You're ok. Just finish up."

I walked out and grabbed my chest. The lady and salesman looked and me and asked if everything was ok. I couldn't talk, I was having a hard time breathing…. and then I started crying. I knew he was ok and he got scared, but the fight response took over and that fear I felt, just got to me.

After my youngest came out of the bathroom. We found his brothers and I broke down again when I told them what happened. My oldest made me sit down. He could tell how upset I was and he wanted to make sure I was going to be ok. My middle son was lecturing my youngest, saying, "you can't scare mom like that because something like that could really hurt her and make her sick. She could die from being scared like that." My youngest didn't see the harm in what he had done, and I wasn't expecting him too.

Having Addison's disease and having a scare like that is never a good thing. My face was going numb and I couldn't slow my heart rate down. My body felt like it had been hit by a truck. I took HC, because stress dosing is always a good idea after something like that.

About an hour later, a horrible flare came on (blurry vision, more numbness in the face, heart palpitations, and shakiness), I was in so much pain and nauseous. The stress that that had caused could have put me in the hospital. I am glad that it didn't. I had to rest after we got home.

It's things like this that really make me hate having Addisons disease. That rise in adrenaline, could have been horrible for me. My body can no longer handle those kinds of scares and we can't prepare for those situations.

******

I remember the first time I got really scared as a mom. My first son was about 10 or 11 months old. He was walking at this time and he didn't want to be held, so I just let him walk. We were at *Ikea* with a friend and we were just enjoying a stroll through the store. Not really looking for stuff but looking at things we wish we could have. I had my eye on him all the time. He wasn't a wanderer and he liked to stay close to me, so I wasn't too worried about him running off, but I still kept a close watch.

My friend was looking at blankets. "Look at this, this one is so soft, and I love the design." I turned and looked "Ya, that is pretty," and then my attention went back down to my son... Who was now gone. My heart sunk, I felt like I couldn't breathe at all. Panic was setting in and I started screaming his name and turning in circles, looking for him.

A man with 2 little girls came up to me, he had my son in his arms. "This one must be yours, because I only have girls" he laughed.

"OMG thank you." I had tears in my eyes.

"We walked past, and he followed my girls."

I laughed. I guess he liked what he saw and decided to follow.

After that, I just carried him. I didn't ever want to let him down.

This happened when I was healthy. It happened, I recovered (within mins), there was no flares, no pain, no scare of, "will this send me to the ER?" I was back to my normal self after a couple mins.

******

Less than a year before I had my back injury, my middle son got sick. I remember calling and talking to my oldest and he told me that his brother had to go to the ER. So, I got on the phone with him and asked him what had happened. He told me that he had told his dad that his penis had swelled up. Well, my ex took that as, *oh he has an erection,* and left it at that. The next day, he told him again, so my ex finally looked. It wasn't only his penis, but his balls, his legs, his hands; he was swelling up. So, they took him to the ER and they gave him some medicine. They said he should be fine in a few days.

I was so mad that my ex didn't even bother to call and tell me. Later that day, my ex called and said they were on their way to a hospital in Tacoma because the swelling was getting worse. I hopped in the car and met them at the hospital.

I was a mess. Not knowing what was going on with my baby. He was so swollen, almost unrecognizable. He was in such good spirits though.

The nurse there was trying to get an IV in him, but they couldn't get it. The nurse kept trying that vein, pushing the needle in and out, over and over again. I was so stressed and pissed at him for trying and failing. My son just laid there, I could tell he was uncomfortable with it, and I finally yelled at the nurse. "Can you please stop. You are not getting it, so please just stop."

He did, and they brought in another nurse. They decided to try the inguinal vein and they were able to get it in quickly. He looked so miserable and it killed me that I couldn't take this pain from him. I wanted whatever was causing him this sickness, to just transfer to me. It's so hard to see your children that sick and there isn't anything you can do about it.

Once they got some fluids in him and some blood work done, they transferred him to a hospital in Bellevue. His kidneys were shutting down for some reason. I was scared. I knew this wasn't good and the Drs. were being so vague about things. I couldn't show him I was scared. I was trying to be brave for him, but when I would leave the room, I would cry.

Once he was in Bellevue, they were able to tell us a bit more. Apparently, he had a case of strep that went undetected (his brother and step sister had strep just a week before) and it started to attack his kidneys.

He was in the hospital for a week. He didn't want me to leave his side at all. I was a mess. Praying that his body would heal. Praying that God wouldn't take him from me.

After a few days of being there and getting the good care that he needed, his nurse came in and said that he was looking pretty good and that most of the swelling had gone down. My son, with a straight face and no emotions said, "except for my penis and balls." We started laughing so hard. I grabbed his little hand and laughed some more. Always such a joker.

Finally, he was discharged. He had to be on a strict diet, so that his kidneys could recover. I was so thankful that he was ok.

This week-long scare was so hard. You never want your kids to be sick and it's so much worse when they are in the hospital and there is nothing you can do.

Looking back, I am thankful that this took place when it did. Being a sick mom, I wouldn't have been able to be around him. With my weak immune system, this could have been fatal for me. I was so thankful that I was there with him. To hold his hand and be there when he needed me most.

******

I always knew that something was off about my youngest. Something changed in him when he was about 3-4 months old. I didn't want to ignore it, but I waited til he was around 1 years old before I made a better observation. He didn't talk, and his first language was ASL. He wasn't like my other boys at all, but he had so much life to him. He was such a happy baby. There were things I noticed about him, that I didn't notice with my other boys.

1) his speech was very delayed. He would say mama, but he was about 13-14 months when he started saying that and it was still not very clear.

2) He would not look you in the eyes at all.

3) Everything had to be routine. If we strayed off his routine, he would have a complete melt down.

4) He was happy to play on his own. Never really engaged much with other kids and when he did, he wasn't sure how to play with them.

When he was about 2 years old. I decided to ask his pediatrician if this was "normal." She set us up with a specialist who determined whether a child is Autistic. I knew that he was. I had worked with Autistic kids in the past. This was not a "scary" thing to me. I knew that even with this diagnosis it wouldn't change how I cared about him, it would only change my perspective of how the world would now treat him….and that scared the hell out of me.

I knew that he would be high functioning. I knew that at some point we would have to deal with bullies, meltdowns, IEPs, and a whole mess of other things. I wanted to be the best mom to him that I could be. I wanted to learn ways to help him excel in life. I would not treat him any different than my older boys, and I would expect the same out of him as I did with them (to an extent).

He got this diagnosis before I was diagnosed with Addisons. I am thrilled about this (let me explain). The stress that some of this had caused, with IEP's and meetings with his teachers, would have sent me into the worst flares (and a couple did, because he was going into 1st grade when I was diagnosed). I feel that I would not have been a great advocate for him at the beginning. I feel that I would have rolled over a lot and let the teachers tell me what needed to be done. One of his teachers wanted to stop giving him homework because it was causing him too much stress. I was not ok with that. I don't expect him to do less because he is Autistic. I expect him to work hard, just like everyone else. I didn't want him to be treated different. He is going to experience stress all his life and it can't just be pushed aside. I felt like they wanted to make this easy for them, so they wouldn't have to deal with him if he had a meltdown.

After homeschooling him (having addisons and fibro), most days I have to stress dose. I wasn't sure how to do that when I was first diagnosed, so this gave me time to figure all that out.

His diagnosis came at right before mine, giving me time to learn and grow with him, and then handle my own diseases while still learning to handle us both.

All kids can stress us out, but this little guy knows that mommy needs him just as much as he needs me. I can't protect him from everything this world will try to do to him, but I know that he has seen the fight in me, and that he will know he is a fighter just like his mom.

******

One of my biggest fears with having Addison's is that it is genetic, and it will be passed on to one of my sons', or some other autoimmune. I know that it's unlikely to happen, but it is still a big fear.

I noticed that my youngest had lost a lot of his energy, so I took him into the naturopath. On July 11, 2018, we got his results back. He was very anemic, which she believes is causing his decline in his energy. His DHEA levels were low as well, and she wasn't sure if that is because of him being so anemic or if it's because his little adrenals are working overtime (also because of the anemia). My heart sank. I was just thinking, *how could I let this happen to him? How could I let his body start to fail him?* but I also gave myself props for recognizing something was off and getting it taken care of.

All we want to do is protect our babies from anything that will harm them, even their own bodies. I never want him to go through what I am going through. It's awful and I wouldn't wish it on anyone. I made sure I got him all the iron, DHEA, and adrenal support supplements asap, so he can give his body a fighting chance. I know that this is going to continue to scare me, to be aware of what his body is doing, and annoy him by asking him a ton of questions about how he is feeling, but I want him as healthy as he can be. I need him to be healthy. He has such an amazing heart and so good at loving people, he needs to share that with the world. I will always be scared for him (for all my boys), but I (for my health), can't stress about it 24/7. All I can do is pray and hope that I can keep them as healthy as I can.

******

One thing that scares me the most is knowing that I might not be around long enough to see my babies get married, have babies, or be successful. I fear that I will miss out on some of the greatest moments of their lives, but what is the worst, is having them lose me too early. How will they handle that? How will they face this world without me when they are not prepared to lose me so early?

I know that it's morbid to think about and anyone can go at any time. Maybe I overreact about it, but I have that right. I am a woman and I am a mom, that is just what we do.

HEALTHY MOM

I was such an active mom. People always asked how I stayed in such great shape…. Have boys. They will keep you busy, on your toes, and running around more than any personal trainer ever could. We went on bike rides, walks, played swords, wrestled, played all the different types of tag, chased each other, danced, ran around, played hide and seek, basketball, soccer, baseball, and all the other things that keep you up and moving. It was very rare that I had a chance to sit down and enjoy peace, but I would not have ever wanted to. My boys are my world and anything they wanted to do with me, I made sure I was up and ready for it.

The only time I really got to rest was when I was in bed with a cold, and even then, we all know what that looks like for a mom. We still have to do all the mom things, just a little slower.

Being able to be so active with them was a joy for me. I have always been an active person and I loved playing sports growing up. I knew that if I had kids, I would make sure they would get to explore whatever sport they possibly could. I wanted them to have a love for it all.

They sure did take advantage of being able to play all the sports and they were/are so amazing at them. Nothing makes me happier than seeing my boys kill it in all their activities.

******

I got my tubes tied when my youngest was just a month old. I didn't have anyone around to help me. I lived about a block from the hospital that I had it done at, so I was lucky enough to be close if anything went wrong. I had been going to a church for a couple months and when I found out when my surgery date was, I asked one of the ladies who I could trust with my 1-month old son, while I went and had this done. There was a sweet teenage girl who watched him for me; free of charge. Thank God, because I didn't have much money at all.

I went in that morning and had it done and was sent home a couple hours later. The girl left as soon as I got home. I was not supposed to lift anything more than 5 lbs. How was I not supposed to lift my baby? I was also breastfeeding…. So, you know what that means…NO PAIN MEDS. Let's just say it was a very, very…VERY… rough couple of days. I had my bed all arranged with diapers, wipes, clothes, garbage sacs (for the diapers), and some food that I could easily shove in my mouth. I got through those days, even though it was one of the hardest things I ever had to do. I was a fucking BOSS!! I don't know how many people could have handled that on their own and I give mad props to all the moms who have had too.

I was healthy, and I got through it. Pain then, doesn't even compare to pain now. Then, I knew it would end. I knew I just had to make it past a couple days and that was it. I would be better, and the pain would be gone. Now, I don't know if it will ever end. I don't know if I will wake up in so much pain that I won't be able to walk. I don't know if I will wake up and have a decent day, but there isn't a day that I don't have pain.

******

My oldest started playing soccer when he was 3 years old. I didn't understand soccer at all. We didn't have it in the town I grew up in and to be honest, I thought it was just something you started to play in college, or if you grew up in Mexico (because it is so big over there). We didn't have it, didn't see it, and didn't watch it. So, I was thrilled when he wanted to play. It gave me a chance to learn another sport. He was such a good player from the get go. He just knew what to do. A little natural athlete. Though he was competitive, he had great sportsmanship.

My middle son, not so much. He didn't like to "compete" as much as my oldest. He liked to pick flowers, twirl around, talk to his teammates, and run up and down the field (not close to the ball). If the ball came at him, he would jump around it. He was so funny to watch. As long as he was having fun, that was all that mattered.

My oldest and I did a 2k family fun run together when he was 7. I had my middle son in his running stroller and before we started the race, I told him that if he needed me to slow down just let me know and I would. We could walk some if he needed too. He had never run this far before, just in soccer games and around our yard. He had asthma, so I made sure I had his inhaler with me just in case he couldn't make it. When the horn went off, he took off like a little rocket. I couldn't catch up with him. After about 3 min, he was gone from my sight. I started to worry that he was going to have an asthma attack. I knew that I might catch up with him. As fast as he was going, he would soon tucker out and have to walk. I was so wrong. He ran the whole way. He ended up coming in 7th place overall with a time of 17 min. He was a beast. I came in around 25 min. I was so proud of him and knew that he was meant to be a runner. He really enjoyed it.

******

We used to go camping. This was so much fun. We would always go to this one camp ground in Eastern Washington. We would stay for about 3 days. The boys were pretty much in the water from sunup til sundown. I would float on the lake on my little innertube floatie thing. I would sometimes go for a run or walk, while they played. Laying out on the shore, taking pics of them having the time of their lives. We would go all day, in the heat, enjoying family time. When it would get dark, we had the fire going, making s'mores, laughing, dancing around. Camping with them was always a blast. In those few days, they would get the best tans ever. They are lucky to be mixed, and they tan really good. I really miss having all the energy to do that.

******

Exercise has always been a big part of my life. Playing sports with the boys, taking them to the park to play soccer or basketball, taking them to workout with me at the gym, going on runs, all the outdoor stuff and workout stuff we could do.

I was always in great shape. I had amazing abs, toned body, I felt great and I looked good. I loved exercising. I know a lot of people hate it, but I fucking love it (still do when I get the chance to). It was a great stress relief for me. I think once you find something that you love, it doesn't seem like you have to work at it, it just makes it more enjoyable. Even though I had some back issues in 2011, I didn't let that stop me from being active with the boys. As painful as it was, I still had the energy to do it.

******

Looking back at my healthy self; I am jealous of her. I miss her. She was fun, fearless, and full of life. She had a blast with her kids and her husband. She could go for miles and never tire. She did everything. She was badass. Working, going out with friends, spending time with her kids, working out, having fun with her husband, having sex, staying out til all hours of the night, drinking (occasionally- I was not a partier), and living her life. She was up for anything and everything. She didn't need sleep, she just needed adventure and fun. She lived a great life. Looking back at all of it, I admire her. She was so strong, even though she felt weak. Even though she had her struggles and hard times, she put on her big girl panties and handled shit. But one day, she couldn't anymore. She was fighting a losing battle. She fought for such a long, long time, but eventually she lost that fight. She had to surrender to her new life. A life that makes her weak and vulnerable. A life that took away what she craved and thrived at. She is a prisoner in a body that tortures her on a daily basis, but is left with all the memories of the person she once was…and can never be again.

STRESSED MOM

We all get stressed as moms…. A LOT. There are so many situations that I could bring up that have caused me so much stress, as a healthy mom and a sick mom. Being a sick mom, it makes these stressful situations a lot harder to deal with, not that I am saying they weren't hard as a healthy mom, I am just saying as a healthy mom, I didn't have to worry about the stress sending me into a crisis that could be fatal.

*****

Graduation for my oldest son was, to say the least, very stressful… and emotional. It really took a toll on my body. It wasn't just the day of his graduation, it was everything leading up to it. The combination of emotions, physical stress, and mental exhaustion hit so hard, but I still had to find it in my to push through.

Back when I was in high school, we had Senior Sunday and graduation… That was it. My son had: Baccalaureate, Senior Signing day (class day), Graduation, and his graduation party. All in the same week. Having to drive for 5 hours (down and back) 3 days in 1 week, with a body that already hates you. That week I was sleeping on a futon because my dad came up early for my son's graduation. In 3 of those days, I only got 9 total hours of sleep. I felt like a zombie but had to function still. I had to plan out the food, make sure the house was clean, got decorations, grocery shopping, cleaning up the yard, answering everyone's questions about the

33

graduation, my mom was calling me and stressing about her dogs having to be alone if she came…. AAAHHHHHH. It hit me hard. I was in so much pain. I was physically, mentally, and emotionally drained…. And the day hadn't even arrived yet.

Of course, I was emotional for all his festivities, but Senior signing day hit me so hard. My son got was crying, so that made me cry even more, but in a good way. I loved seeing him get emotional about his time with his friends and what they had to say during speeches and him tearing up over seeing baby pictures of himself. It really made me proud.

I wasn't sure how to prepare for how many people were going to come (I forgot to have them RSVP-so I had no clue how many would actually show up). We invited 100 guests, so I figured about 50 people would come. I overprepared, but it is always better to overprepare than underprepare. I was able to send food (and lots of it) home with guests. The boys took some food down to their dad's house as well. I got rid of all the food that I didn't need/want in the house, so it was a win/win for everyone.

I enjoyed/hated this time. I am pretty sure I overdosed a bit on ibuprofen, just to get through it (not that it helped a lot). I was sad that it was over and he was done with his high school career. He would be going off to college soon and I am not sure if I am ready for that. But, I was also glad for it to be done so I could have some rest. As a mom… does that word even exist for us?

******

Being a healthy mom, was easier for me (obviously). From 2007-2010 I was a single mom. That was a very interesting time. Trying to make ends meet at shitty jobs, was not easy. I tried to spend as much time as I could with the boys, yet having to work 2-3 jobs and going to school full time; it was fucking stressful. I was able to do it though. I had the energy, I was go-go-go constantly, but I got shit done.

Looking back at those times, I don't know how I did it (by the grace of God). I would wake up early, go to bed late, work, do school work, workout/run, make it to my kid's games, take them out to play in parks, and still held it together.

Being sick, I can no longer do that. I have to use my "spoons" carefully. Somedays I have enough energy to get up, get dressed, and that's it. Somedays I can clean the house, make it to appointments, and games, but then I am paying for the next couple days. I am on the couch and can barely get myself up to use the bathroom.

How do I not look at myself as a failure?

I know that this isn't my fault. I didn't ask to have Addisons Disease and Fibromyalgia. I just always thought I would be healthy and be able to do everything I wanted to do. This was not the life I wanted.

Stress is now something I have to avoid. I laugh at this because, how the fuck do you avoid stress and still try to have somewhat of a "normal" life. I have 3 boys and a husband….

How do I avoid stress? I don't. I can't. It's not like it's something you can see coming your way. It happens, and I just try to minimize it when I can. Does it cause me to have flares? Yes. Has stress sent me into a crisis?

Yes, a few times. But here I am, still alive, and dealing with this life the best way I can.

There is not magic cure for dealing with stress. If there is…. Please let me know.

You just have to learn how to deal with it, to minimize its effect on you, and let your family and friends know that they need to keep their drama far away from you, because the way if affects them, could be more fatal to you.

******

One of the first times I realized that stress really affected my Addisons was back in November 2014. I was driving the older two boys down to drop them off at their dads. I don't know why it stressed me out, but it did. I noticed that I started to have some numbness on the right side of my face, and it had come and gone throughout the day, when I would think about having to see their dad. It didn't last too long, but I was doing better at tracking my symptoms since I was newly diagnosed. I wanted to be aware of what my body was doing. This numbness, thinking back, had been there before (when I had to deal with him), but I never really noticed, or cared to notice it.

My ex and his wife can cause me the biggest stress. I almost always have to stress dose when I am about to see them. Sometimes when we are at an event, they will all out ignore me when I ask a question. Or they will give me dirty looks. Literally they will look at me like I am trash. Yet, on social media she will act like she is the nicest person ever and that she cares.

That stresses me the fuck out. I want things to be good with us, and Lord knows I have tried. I don't want it to be awkward for my kids. We are fucking adults. We should be able to handle getting along. For some reason, when we are in person, they just can't seem to give me the time of day.

It really makes me sad for the boys. I feel that they feel awkward about it and they shouldn't. It's been 11 years. We should be over whatever issues we've had by now. I will continue to try. I will continue to be nice, but it stresses me out.

******

Having to get ready to go out with friends is a huge stress. I don't have much of an immune system. I don't have a lot of energy to put into making myself look nice. I don't have the energy to last long while I am out either. On my good days, it is a lot easier, but I also want to use my good days to get shit done around my house (to get the shit done that I have been putting off because I had zero spoons). I don't want to waste those spoons on going out with my friends. I know, I sound like a shitty friend, but it's true.

I mostly always go, unless it is a really bad day. One of the last times I went out, I was so exhausted, it wasn't even enjoyable. I feel like I was a buzz kill. That is not fun for my friends. I feel that it makes it hard for them to have a good time, and that is not fair to them. I love when we just hang out at one another's houses. That is a lot easier. I know I can fall asleep or lounge on their couches and not be judged. I don't want to have to stress about going out in public. I don't even like people. It's not fun for spoonies to be out. People are sick, people touch you, people are annoying. I don't like being around that.

I am so thankful my friends are very understanding of my situation. They will invite me to all the stuff, but they don't get pissy or mad if I turn them down or bail at the last minute. They are here for me when I need them. Even though I try not to stress about going out with them…. I still stress.

******

Have you ever had to travel? Packing for yourself and your children? What does your spouse do? This is such a stress for me when we get ready to go on vacations, camping, and overnight stays. I have to make sure I pack enough for everyone. I have to make sure all the meds are packed, toothbrushes, deodorant, extra clothes (just in case my ASD child has an accident), medical supplies (because I have 3 very active boys), all the toiletries, snacks, etc…. My husband throws shit in a bag and calls it good. He doesn't stress about all the things we will need.

Traveling already hurts my body. Sleeping in hotels hurts my body. Standing or sitting too long hurts my body. But I love to see how happy my kids are, having a good time; the pain is worth the memories; the flares are worth the smiles. My kids enjoy when we all go out together and do things as a family. They see that it takes a toll on me, only after we get home and I allow myself to fall apart from it.

I don't want to ruin their fun by having them see me sick. I want them to have great memories. But the stress of having to hide all of it, just makes the pain worse. I know they love me so much and that they want me to rest and to not push myself, but if that was the case, I would never leave home and those would not be the memories I would want them to have.

******

Having a son on the spectrum is STRESSFUL!!!! He is a joy most of the time, but OMFG this kid can throw you for a loop. He is so wonderfully weird and everywhere we go I worry for him. When we are at a playground, lake, sporting events; I worry kids will be mean to him (as we all do as parents, not just with the kids with disabilities).

One day we were at the lake and he was being pushed off the dock by these 3 teenage girls (about 13-14 years old). They were pushing other kids off too. They were bigger girls, expressing their dominance or whatever the fuck they thought they were doing, but this time, they were messing with the wrong kid. When he was trying to get back on the dock, they would push him back in. I saw that he was swimming away and it looked like he was trying to stop himself from crying. I got his attention and motioned him to come out of the water and talk to me. When I asked him what was wrong, he looked at the dock and shrugged his shoulders. I asked him again and he was holding back tears. I laid his towel out for him to sit on and said, "talk to me, let me know what is going on." He started crying and telling me what the girls had done. The mama bear in me wanted to storm over there and shove those little fucking brats into the water and ask them "how do you like being shoved by someone bigger and older?"
I let him collect himself and told him that I was going to go on the dock with him and he could jump off if he wanted to. He was reluctant, but I

told him that I would be right there with him, so he didn't have anything to worry about. At this point my face was starting to get numb, so I knew I was stressing. I was fucking pissed at how these girls were acting. Where were their parents? Did their parents even care that they were targeting smaller kids and being bullies? I wasn't sure what I was going to say to these girls, or what I was going to do. I knew that I couldn't lay a hand on them (as much as I wanted to). I am an adult and I needed to act as such. As we walked down the dock, the girls were looking at me. They knew that I was coming straight at them. They looked nervous AF. I walked up to them, and I was close enough that I could have wrapped my hand around the back of the girl's head (don't worry. I didn't). I just looked at them and calmly said, "You lay a hand on my son again, you and I are going to have a problem." (I think it is scarier when you calmly threaten someone). The girls' eyes got really wide and all they said was "OK." I smiled, turned, and walked back to where I was sitting. They didn't push any other kids off the dock after that.

When I got back to my seat, my whole right side of my face was so numb. My heart was beating really fast, I swear you could hear it, I was short of breath and shaking. Talk about stress-pissed, I knew this could be a moment that I would need to take some extra hydrocortisone. I was definitely feeling the Addisons.

I kept a close watch on the girls, and noticed they kept looking at me as well. I saw that my youngest had stopped and talked to them after he had jumped in a few times. He came back and told me they were being nice to him. I love that even though they were horrible, he found it in his heart to not hold a grudge. That he wanted to still be friends with them. That made my mommy heart fill up and over flow.

******

I stress about stresses that I should not be stressing about, but it's so stressful with all the shit that runs through my head. I play things out in about 100 different ways, and most of those scenarios never even happen. I have conversations with myself, what I will say to people, what will happen if I go out to the grocery store and run into someone I know but don't want to talk to…. Which 99% of the time NEVER HAPPENS. But for some reason, it's going on in my head, and causing me to stress. FOR NO REASON.

I honestly don't know why I do this. I am sure you do this too. It's not fun. Maybe it's boredom or maybe misery loves company…. Who knows why we put ourselves through this.

I always tell myself, "don't stress out. Don't let this affect you." Do I listen… Nope. Do I love drama. FUCK NO!! So why do I have to stress about things that are never going to happen?? Is it because, as a woman, we are built to do this? Who knows, but I don't like it. I really need to learn to stop doing it. Shit, I stress about this book, writing it, editing it, publishing it. The never-ending cycle of stress.

NEWLY DIAGNOSED MOM

Several months before I was diagnosed, I felt like I had no energy. My body was failing me in every way. I wasn't as vibrant and active as I use to be. I wasn't getting the answers I needed from the doctors. I wasn't going to believe that I was just "getting old" and that this was going to be my life from now on. I have 3 active boys and a young husband. I didn't have time to feel fatigued for no reason. I knew that with my back being so bad, that could have caused some of the fatigue. My body was fighting pain daily, but still, it was something that I had dealt with before, so this shouldn't be new.

When I had my surgery in December of 2011, I remember they had a hard time with me breathing after receiving anesthesia, so I had to stay in the hospital for a few days until that passed. My surgeon and nurses thought that was a little strange, but we didn't think much of it at the time. It wasn't normal, but it wasn't something that I was concerned about either.

My primary Dr. had just told me that I was getting old and these were just the symptoms of that. She was the Dr., with a degree, so she must see this all the time…. Right? But, I just couldn't believe it, because none of my friends were going through this, so why was I.

When I finally said, fuck you to my quack of a Dr. I went and saw a Naturopath. A friend of mine told me to check out this one place in Mukilteo, so I did. I looked at the Naturopaths available, picked one, and made an appointment. I was a little nervous because I wasn't sure what to expect. I had been battling with bronchitis for about a couple months now, and I wanted to get that checked out as well, but wasn't sure what a naturopath could do for that.

The office was very nice, lots of natural light, everything was white. It was almost like something out of a movie. The nurse called me back and did my weight and took my vitals. So far, it was just like a normal Dr. appointment, nothing weird, nothing uncomfortable.

As I waited for the naturopath to come in, my youngest was bouncing all over the room. I was trying to keep him under control but was having a hard time.

She came in and was so nice. She asked me lots of questions and I answered them, told her all my symptoms and how I had bronchitis that wouldn't go away. I told her about my back surgery, and how this all could play a part in my exhaustion, and then said, "You know, everything that comes with getting older." She smiled at me and said "at your age, no. This is not symptoms of getting older."

I did a nervous laugh. She was typing things out on her laptop. "I want to do some bloodwork. From what you are telling me, I think that you might have Addison's Disease."

"Oh. Ok." I said. Like I knew what Addisons Disease was.

"Have you heard of it before?"

"No." I said. I didn't even know what to ask about it. I was just not expecting to have anything.

"JFK had it." She said, and I shook my head, waiting for a better description of it. "When I was going to school to be a naturopath, one of the girls in my class had it. It's when your adrenal glands are not working. Your adrenals produce cortisol and with Addisons, they don't. I want to do blood work to make sure that is what this is and see how all your other levels look as well, then we can go from there."

We talked a bit more about other things, but my brain was just focusing on what this might mean for my life. I wasn't sure what it was, but I also didn't want to ask too many questions. The nurse came in a took some blood and then I talked more with the Naturopath. She didn't seem to want me to leave until I felt comfortable with what she had told me and if there were any other concerns she could help me with. I felt pretty good when I left, for the most part. Now it was just a waiting game. She said she would call when the results from the bloodwork came back, but to set up an appointment so we can go over them together. I didn't realize that I had been with her for almost 2 hours. I have never been to a doctor who took that much time with their patients. It was nice to not have to be rushed so they can move onto the next one.

I scheduled my next appointment for the following week and went on my way. I, of course, googled what Addisons Disease was, what affect it would have on me, and how it would change my life. I didn't do much research on it. I was pretty happy with the results I found in my first search. It didn't sound bad. I would just have to take a couple pills a day and I would be good to go. I was thankful it wasn't anything serious… So I thought at the time.

When I went back the following week and the results had confirmed that I indeed had Addisons Disease. I told her I googled it and was thankful it wasn't serious. She looked at me very confused. "This is something to take very seriously."

From what I read, it didn't sound bad, but from her reaction… I knew that it wasn't good. She told me a bit more about it. How I would have to avoid people who are sick, because my immune system would be weak and probably why I can't kick the bronchitis. She mentioned that I would have to take steroids for the rest of my life to replace what my adrenals weren't producing. And that I need to avoid getting stressed and to not get into any accidents and that type of stuff, because it could cause my body to go into an adrenal crisis, which can be fatal.

All this info was a bit much. I didn't get that far into researching it. It didn't seem so scary coming from google, but it was a horror movie coming from her. She gave me a referral to an endocrinologist, who I would have to see every 3-4 months, probably for the rest of my life. I left feeling a little lost. I really didn't know what any of this meant. I was scared, knowing that a common cold could kill me. Stress could kill me. All these new things I would have to learn to take care of my body to make sure that I could function. It was all overwhelming.

In my first year of being diagnosed with Addisons disease, it was quite an eye opener. I didn't realize a big change until I started really listening to my body and paying attention to what it was doing. I wanted to journal, so I could look back and figure out what caused bad days and what caused good days.

Journal Entry: November 2014-December 2015

November 3, 2014:
No symptoms today- Energy throughout the day. Tired around 9pm. Good day.

November 4, 2014:
Very good day again-lots of energy-out of bed by 8:30am.

Tired around 7pm. Hope for more days like this.

November 5, 2014:
Another good day- No symptoms, though I feel myself getting sick. I don't feel tired right now at 11:35pm, but I hope I won't struggle with insomnia. Would be nice to have another good sleep.
Just hope I don't get sick. I don't have time for a cold right now.

November 7, 2014:
YAY! Another great day. Loving this. I feel like I got meds under control. Yesterday I did have the fast potties, but that was it.
I love the energy I have and that I am actually tired at night.
Waiting for a crash though. Hopefully not, but we will see.

December 17, 2014:
Felt very symptomatic. Numbness, dizziness, nausea, blurry vision, body pain, and headache.

December 18, 2014:
Worse than yesterday. Very dizzy and nauseous. I don't like where this is going. I don't know if I am sick or if this is stress related, but I don't feel right.

December 19, 2014:
Went to ER. Everything was fine. Stress from not knowing when I was getting the boys caused me to have an adrenal crisis. This was my first crisis and I had no clue what was going on. I felt weak, dizzy, nauseous, lethargic, and pain throughout my body. I didn't know what was going on, but I was really scared. I didn't want to go to the hospital and I put it off. I finally got to the point where I was looking so bad, that my husband forced me to go. I am so glad he did. I can't ignore this stuff. I have to start taking this disease seriously. I could have wound up in a coma or something worse. They gave me an IV of fluids and some HC and then sent me on my way when my vitals looked good.

The nurse that I had there, had been a nurse for 22 years and I am the 2nd patient she had seen with Addison's disease (it had been about 15 years in-between). I was shocked that the Dr. didn't really know what it was and I am pretty sure he googled it. That didn't really make me feel great about him treating me. Hopefully I won't ever have another one again.

I do wonder if I do happen to have another one, will it be the same symptoms?

December 26, 2014:

Went to Endo. Starting me on aldosterone replacement. Did blood tests and a 24-hour urine monitoring.

Started monitoring BP and HR.

7:17pm- Boys being rambunctious. Was mildly stressed 101/65 HR 67

10:46pm- After showering. 104/54 HR 69

11:16pm- Resting for 20 min-Error 1st taken- laying down 92/49 HR 61

Standing up quickly after 11:17pm- 107/70 HR 97

Sitting down quickly after 11:19pm- 103/59 HR 68

Yesterday deep pain, like my muscles were about to spasm in my glutes. Had my husband massage my L. side. Tonight, pain (like growing pains) in my L. leg all the way to my feet. Almost hurts to walk. Little dizzy today. Very tired, felt like I needed a nap around 3pm.

Dr. altered my hydrocortisone. 2 when I wake up and 1 four hours later and 1 before dinner. I can't get the fludrocortisone til Monday.

Gonna start urine 24-hour collection on Monday night so I can take it in Wednesday morning or Saturday night so they can have it Monday morning.

December 27, 2014:

Took BP about 10 min after a massage at 11:04am 98/69 HR 54

Took when I felt exhausted and needed a nap. 3:47pm 98/62 HR 60

In bed- annoyed at my brother and the boys. 9:41pm 86/49 HR 60

Felt really exhausted today. Took a nap for about an hour. Kind of irritable today. Felt short on patience.

Had a massage in the morning and felt good after. No body aches in the low back or legs, but my left neck/shoulder area was achy.

Started my 24-hour pee collection at 9:27am. Filled 1 container already. Such a pain to do. Cannot wait for it to be over.

Kind of nervous to start the new meds just because of the side effects and having my immune system shot. I am anxious about all the blood tests and what they were for and their results. What if I have something other than Addisons???

I am noticing a big difference when my youngest has gluten. He is so hyper and out of control. He can't control his body at all and is super crazy. I really need to go to the gluten free store and get him everything he needs. I want him to be able to control himself.

Getting worried that the boys won't make it to *Great Wolf Lodge*. I feel that my oldest is choosing sports over family-which is not good. I don't know how to talk with him about it without making him feel pressured. I hate being away from them so much, but I feel they really don't care about being away from me at all. Do I just let them come up when they want, or keep set weekends just to be disappointed when they don't come? I just wish it was easier. I wish they could see how it affects my Addisons and all the symptoms I go through.

No one understands, and I feel like I'm complaining all the time and that even talking about it annoys people. I really need an outlet and answers and energy.

10:06pm 94/61 HR 65

December 28, 2014:
Waking up at 9:09am 96/63 HR 79
Getting ready to take boys back. Feeling ok, light dizziness.
12:28pm 99/67 HR 73
Driving home. Face started to feel numb
3:02pm 99/62 HR 70
Feeling super exhausted like I need a nap.
4:38pm 125/61 HR 70
4:39pm 109/71 HR 71
So tired all day. Crawled into bed at 8pm. Hard time keeping my eyes open. Hoping for a better day tomorrow.

The boys went back today. I pray that my ex lets them come for the weekend. All I want is to have a good relationship with him for the boys, but I feel his wife has a lot to do with why we don't. All I can do is pray. In bed 8:09pm 97/60 HR 72

December 29, 2014:
Again, around 12:30pm felt extremely tired. Took a nap and felt better. After my nap: 3:25pm 99/65 HR 80
Felt pretty good the rest of the day. Got my meds and found out they will make me gain a bunch of weight, mostly water weight, but still not a good sign.

December 30, 2014:
Waking up 10am 83/51 HR 54
Was up til 3:30am texting with a friend and taking quizzes online. My body needs sleep. Woke up not very tired though. So that is a plus. I need to get a lot done today but have to take my youngest with me, so that is going to be an adventure.
Missed getting to see a friend from out of state this morning. I haven't seen her in so long.
Weighed myself this morning with clothes on (138.6lbs) Took BP late afternoon after being lazy all day. 5:25pm 93/59 HR 60

December 31, 2014:
After being awake and lying in bed for an hour- 9:54am 84/51 HR 51
Sitting up 9:56am 80/54 HR 79
Standing up 9:59am 97/56 HR 106
Weight in the am 138.2 lbs. 11:51am 110/65 HR 80

January 1, 2015:
After a long night of drinking and sleeping til 1pm. 1:30pm 105/62 HR 80
Had a lot of fun last night. Drank too much as usual. Glad I just get to lay in bed all day. I'm super exhausted, but I think I need lazy days like this.

Weighed myself after my shower- 139lbs at 2pm.

3:27pm 79/55 HR 79

Lying in bed for a few hours and then moving around for a bit 5:14pm 100/68 HR 70

Took my youngest to see *Big Hero 6*. Really great movie, not what I had expected, but loved the movie. He did really good in the theater, which was really nice for a change.

Headed to bed 10:15pm 96/61 HR 69

January 2, 2015:

Feeling tightness in my head, neck, and into my chest. 11:54am- 104/65 HR 101

Heading to bed after relaxing for a bit. 12:12am 107/66 HR 79

Same weird tightness in neck, shoulders, and chest. Not the same feeling of tightness that I have had before. Strange. Thought maybe it was my neck needing an adjustment or tight muscles, but it went away during the day, but came back later in the night. Watched my friend's little ones for a few hours. Love having the baby, but not sure I actually would be able to do that all over. I feel bad for my husband. I want to be able to do this for him, but not sure I can handle a new born all over again, especially with how tired I am already.

January 5, 2015:

BP after working out and cool down stretch. 3:40pm 99/67 HR 113

Went to *Great Wolf Lodge* for the weekend. Had tightness in the back of my head, into my jaw and down into my chest. Could hardly take a breath. Scared me really bad. It's happened every day since Saturday. Slowly getting back into working. Really missed work. Really fatigued today, need a nap. Cleaned kitchen 6:43 106/62 HR 118

January 6, 2015:

Lying in bed til 11:33am 99/73 HR 80

Ran out of my meds yesterday. Not sure when I will be able to get them refilled. Worked out for the 1st time yesterday in what seems like forever.

I'm so out of shape, but ready to kick my body back into gear and make it part of my lifestyle.

Finally got a call that my meds were in. The pharmacist asked why I am on both and to talk with my Dr. about that. Apparently she knows nothing about Addisons disease.

Craft night was finally back on. We all have sewing machines, so it's time to start making some clothes and getting better at it.

January 7, 2015:

Waking up 10:30am 83/54 HR 60

After my workout and 1 min cool down 1:39pm 91/67 HR 147

January 8, 2015:

Kind of a lazy day. Weighed myself in the am and I was 137 lbs. So happy I haven't gained weight like the pharmacist said.

Took a rest day from working out. Hopefully I can keep up the progress.

Nice to have the house semi to myself.

Feeling like I am going to blow up at my oldest brother any min. I am going to have to lay down some strict rules to help us save money.

My husband got a call from his old boss, but never called him back. That is one thing that really bugs me about him is his lack of follow through; stresses me out so much. I know he would get annoyed if someone didn't call him back- kind of like how he was with the Union guy who didn't call him back. Just pick up the phone, goodness. AAAHHHH!!!!

I don't know how long I've been bugging him about the light outside. I don't care if we are behind in rent, just get stuff done. I don't even know if he's done anything with our taxes yet. But somehow, I get blamed for putting things away where he can't find them-excuse me it's right there on our desk. Move shit around and look or better yet…. ASK!!

10:04pm 97/64 HR 61

Didn't feel like I needed a nap today, but I did have low energy.

Not as sore, but still feeling it, especially in the low back. Getting back into it tomorrow and pushing myself.

January 9, 2015:

Waking up-sitting up 88/65 HR 90 @ 10:57am

Started feeling dizzy and light headed. 3:45pm 108/66 HR 80

Crawled into bed-down for the night 9:16pm 97/61 HR 81

Finally told my older brother no more pot in the house. He got upset and went to his room. I was so mad I was shaking. I'm so fed up with him and his child like behavior. I'm trying to make him so upset so he can finally get a fire under his ass and move out.

Pretty exhausted today. I wanted to take a nap, but I got a workout in and that felt great. Looking forward to one tomorrow, just have to fit it in between my clients or before my first client.

Heard from my Dr. and he said that my cortisol levels are looking good with the cortisol hormones I am taking, but there are things he needs to discuss with me about my other results. I hate having to wait so long for results. I just want answers. I really need to see a counselor. I can't handle all these emotions that I can't let out. I just want to scream.

My husband had his Union meeting and his old boss wants to hire him back. Big decisions to make, hopefully he won't have a freak out (night terrors) with all this on his plate. I need to sleep, and I need him to make the right decisions for us, because I don't even know what to tell him.

January 11, 2015:

After no sleep last night and being up with my youngest vomiting 12:31pm 103/62 HR 86

Got a Thai massage which was very centering. I really enjoyed it. Less stress today.

January 12, 2015:

I got 4 hours of sleep in the past 36 hours. I am so exhausted. Off to see my Endocrinologist again today. Hopefully everything will be all balanced out and the meds will start working, or if they are already working. Dr. thinks that when I get stressed my heart isn't pumping the right amount of blood needed, so that's why I get the heaviness and dizziness. Adjusting my fludro to 1 ½ pills and going to do a spit test to see my cortisol levels at night. Hoping to lower it so I can sleep. He says my BP is still way to low.

My oldest brother didn't come out of his room til 11:45am and then he yelled at my youngest for being loud while he is resting. I'm no longer gonna have him help with him anymore if this behavior continues. This is ridiculous.

January 14, 2015:

10:37am 93/60 HR 80.

Finally got some sleep last night after only getting like 8 hours in a 60-hour period. It wasn't the best sleep, but I feel more rested today. Got a run/walk in today. Great to have an escape. Was nice to get out of the house yesterday too.

Worked out, stretched, showered, got laundry done, and kitchen cleaned. Got some alone time which was so nice.

2:59pm 101/70 HR 99

Took my youngest to dance class and went to get him his gluten free snacks. Today his teacher told me he tried to cut a girl's hair. Crazy kid. He thought it would look better short. I would hate to meet with the mom if he had gone through with it.

10:21pm 100/58 HR 79

Talked to a friend of a friend who has Addisons and she is worried about my health, because I'm always bordering on having a crisis. No one understand how scary this is, so I am so glad I was able to find her.

If I don't see better results with my Dr. I will switch to the guy she is seeing.

It's like every day I can feel anxiety and that scares me. What if I get so upset it puts me in the hospital? What if I don't get to say goodbye to the boys? I wish I had people close who understood how serious this really is. My middle brother does, and he is trying to get me to slow down, which I need too, but I feel like I have to be on hyperdrive all the time.

Adjusted the time on my hydrocortisone to 5pm. I felt that helped last night. BP is looking pretty good the last couple days. Tonight, I took Benadryl and melatonin to see if I can get some good sleep. My husband dropped off his truck tonight at his work and starts work with his old boss tomorrow. Hopefully this will be the last job change for a few years.

Haven't heard from the boys in about a week. Definitely taking their phones away. They really need to know that I am serious about getting a hold of me. Especially with how I am. Would help lower my stress if they contacted me more.

January 15, 2015:
Feeling dizzy 1:44pm 105/76 HR 97
Extremely tired and dizzy 3:01pm 97/62 HR 81
Had a burst of energy today. Cleaned the living room, vacuumed, cleaned and vacuumed the car. Then I got a rush of fatigue. Hard to keep eyes open, feeling of being dizzy/buzzed. Thought I was having a good day, but that went away pretty quickly.

January 16, 2015:
8:56am 90/55 HR 60
After talking with my ex 10:23am 97/69 HR 90
Needing a nap 4:22pm 96/61 HR 74
Took my youngest to the dentist to get his teeth pulled since the bottom 2 adult teeth came in. He handled it really good. Took him out to get a treat after. He also has gone 3 nights without peeing his diaper, which is so great. I'm so proud of him.
Talked with my ex today and my oldest is going on a ride along with him tonight. I'm super nervous about it, but I know he will be fine.
My middle son has a tournament this weekend that we won't be able to make it to. I hate having to miss all his games. I just can't travel as much anymore. I'm missing out on so much.
I just want to escape. I want some time away to "play" for myself and relax and lay in bed and watch *F.R.I.E.N.D.S.*

January 17, 2015:
Drama last night after our friend's party, but glad it all got sorted out. Our friend has some major self-esteem issues and is crushing on a guy who doesn't like her, and any attention he gives to someone else, she accuses them of trying to get with him. In this case it was me. She was accusing us of having an affair. All I did was give this guy a ride. She tried to convince

my husband that we were having an affair. Sorry, girl. Don't have time for your crazy.

My husband talked about how me not wanting a baby really bothers him and he is just trying to process it all. I want him to be able to have what he wants; he just can't have it with me. I think time apart for us is a really good thing.

Laid in bed all day and took a 2 ½ hour nap.

7:40pm 105/64 HR 67

January 18, 2015:

Stayed the night at a friend's last night. Was so nice to get away and have a good night's rest and some girl time.

Came home and did laundry and cleaned the kitchen.

Things between my husband and I are still weird, not sure how long this will last, but I just can't be physical with him right now. I think once my brothers are gone it will be easier for us to talk and work things out, but until then, this whole situation has me under so much stress. Being with/around him is just too much. I really don't want to be touched at all.

9:31pm 102/52 HR 70. Got to get my bottom number in the 60's.

January 19, 2015:

Let my youngest sleep in just underwear last night and he stayed dry. So proud of him. He is growing up so fast.

10:11am 109/59 HR 79

Didn't sleep well last night. My husband kept moving, talking, snoring, and tossing then little man came in at 5am. I need my own bedroom.

12:06pm 106/73 HR 81

After doing 30 min workout-cardio, legs, thighs, and butt @12:55pm 99/69 HR 128

January 21, 2015:

Ran around all day. Dropped my oldest brother off at his appointment.

Took my youngest to school, got my hair dyed and trimmed, picked up my brother, got my youngest from school, went to my Dr., came home, made dinner, visited with a friend, bath, and bed.

8:15pm 89/52 HR 71

Had some dizziness today. My oldest brother said he is making it a priority to move out, which is taking a huge burden and weight off my shoulders. I just want my house back and my home life to be peaceful.

I don't know what to do about my husband still. I feel things are changing and that I'm just wanting to let go, just to give him his desire to have a child with someone else. IDK if he has anyone to talk to about it, but I don't know what else to do.

9:36pm 96/64 HR 61

January 23, 2015:

Needing sleep. So hard to get sleep at night and with my youngest coming in and waking me up at 6am, just makes it really hard.

11:18am 105/64 HR 79

I hate being so stressed out that I don't even want to be in my own home. Hopefully my oldest brother will be out soon.

Trying to discipline youngest and not agreeing with my husband. My oldest brother thinks he needs to chime in and co-parent. I got this. I don't need help. Super frustrating.

Eating dinner, my stomach pain was so bad I could only eat a little. Felt really sick, like I am going to vomit.

6:49pm 123/71 HR 66

7:22pm 91/55 HR 60

January 24, 2015:

Drove down to Tacoma to watch my oldest son play. He is now slightly taller than me; my baby boy is growing so fast. I miss them so much. Hurts my heart not being able to see them as much. Christmas was the last time they came up to stay with us.

Can't wait for my brothers to move out and I can start getting my house back to normal. Just trying to decide what to do with the spare room. Keep it an extra room? Turn it into a workout room? Have it as a game room for the boys? Gotta start figuring it out so I can plan.

I need a massage so bad. I'm hurting. Can't wait for my craniosacral on Tuesday just to help kind of level me out a bit.

January 25, 2015:
11:18am 103/65 HR 79
12:46pm 98/61 HR 118
8:26pm 106/63 HR 69

Went and visited with a friend today. Nice to see her since it's been almost a year since we saw each other last. My youngest didn't handle the visit well. Her youngest daughter upset him a few times and her oldest daughter doesn't share well, but he still had fun.
I passed out on the couch around 7pm for an hour. Heading to bed early tonight. I'm super exhausted.

January 26, 2015:
11:42am 107/60 HR 67
6:05pm 96/64 HR 70

Got a workout in after missing Saturday and Sunday. I'm still sore from Friday's workout, but it's good that I'm staying on track. Just have to get my husband on board. Wondering if I wake up with him in the morning and we workout together, if he will be more inclined to actually working out. He needs to do something. I think when he gets paid I need to plan out healthy meals and change something so that will help him as well.
Finally feeling that my hair growth is progressing. Feels like it's been this long for a year.
2 clients today. Really wishing things would pick up soon. I want to not struggle financially in our personal and business. It's hard when we are supporting the 5 of us and 2 other adults.
Got to figure out a way to do some better marketing and keep clients coming in regularly.

January 28, 2015:
11:41am 92/63 HR 73
10:25pm 96/57 HR 64

Worked out, deep conditioned hair, watched one of my shows, slow boring day.

January 29, 2015:

Full day at the office. Actually had some energy today.

7:08pm 122/66 HR 73

Stayed at the office for some much needed me time. Was so nice. I need to do that more often.

I shouldn't feel like I don't want to go back to my own home, but the stress is too much on me right now. I am not handling it well, but I am at a loss of what to do.

February 2, 2015:

My team won yesterday. YAY Patriots. So much fun hanging out with friends. Super Bowl Champs!

8:52pm 115/70 HR 68

Meds are finally working for my BP. Which is great. Now if I can only get the energy I need.

Last night was really rough with my youngest, so tonight I did the benytonin cocktail (Benadryl and melatonin) so I can sleep and hopefully my husband will get up with him.

I'm so exhausted. Just want some energy and sleep.

Having time to myself and getting out more has certainly helped with my stress levels. So nice to not be around the chaos that I call home.

I miss the boys so much. Been a long time since I've seen them. Hoping they miss me just as much.

February 3, 2015:

Slept amazing last night. I really needed that.

8:45am 100/67 HR 68

Fell asleep around 8:45pm. Woke up about 4 times but only for a couple mins, then slept really good til about 5:30am when little man came in.

I feel really rested this morning.

12:10pm 109/62 HR 79

February 5, 2015:
Got 4 hours of sleep last night.
9:28am 114/68 HR 79

February 6, 2015:
Laying down. 9:01am 98/54 HR 54
Standing 9:03am 97/60 HR 102
Sitting 9:04am 99/60 HR 65
Slept pretty good last night and went to bed early (for me) and enjoyed some alone time watching shows and listening to music.
Went and napped at my office. Really needed that.
Today seems super stressful. Lots of tightness in my chest.
4:36pm 97/60 HR 91

February 7, 2015:
Long day at the office. Came home and napped for 2 hours.
10:27pm 116/65 HR 80
Super exhausted. Hopefully I can get rest tonight. I need sleep so bad.
Drank 2 Angry Orchards tonight and I am super tired and slightly drunk. More like 1 and a couple drinks from the 2nd. We will see if I can even finish it.

February 8, 2015:
11:06am 69/61 HR 69
Slept bad last night. My youngest coming in is really hard to deal with. My husband's snoring is hard to deal with. I am definitely making the extra room, my bedroom. I need more sleep.
My husband just kicked the ball out from under my youngest and he got hurt. Why would he think that's a good idea?
12:35pm 98/61 HR 73
2:34pm 92/59 HR 74
I hate feeling how I feel. I hate avoiding everyone. Especially when I just want to spend time with my youngest and he is all over everyone else. I can't wait to have time when it's just me and the boys.

8:39pm 97/61 HR 59

Cleaned the house today. Feeling really irritable today. I know I'm starting my period in a couple days. My stomach has been a bit crampy today. Kinda want to get on BC so I don't have to have my period anymore. I've been feeling yucky lately. Feeling like I should start doing my make-up and hair again, dressing better. Maybe that would help me feel better. I think I'm getting too comfortable not looking nice or I'm just looking old now.

February 10, 2015:

10:51am 113/61 HR 65

10:04pm 98/59 HR 79

I hate staying in my bed all morning, so I don't have to deal with homelife. I want it to be me and the boys. I think it's hard because it's been so long since I have been able to see them. I want my brothers out, more my oldest then the middle one. I want our house back, I want to be in love again with my husband (not that I fell out of love), I want to want him, I want him to lose weight and actually want to have a better body. I want him to see a Dr. about his snoring and night terrors so I can sleep better at night. I am thankful that he is a wonderful father to my boys though.

I need some help. I just want to be happy, energetic and full of life again.

February 11, 2015:

11:16am 98/70 HR 73

3:01pm 99/65 HR 79

So, the Dr. appointment happened today. He is upping my fludro by half a pill. Lowering my hydro by half a pill and wants me to wear a heart monitor for 24 hours to see if I have a heart issue. He thinks something might be off with my pituitary gland too. I'm all sorts of a hot mess.

February 12, 2015:

12:43 104/68 HR 79

Worked a full day. 4 clients is a lot to take on for me. I'm exhausted and I know that I won't sleep.

7:57pm 99/63 HR 80

Heart palp after I took my BP. Enough to take my breath away. Almost feels like someone is squeezing my heart.

Got to talk to my good friend from Iowa for a couple hours today, that was really nice.

February 13, 2015:

My youngest stayed in his bed all night. I slept all night, but I am super exhausted.

10:17am 110/67 HR 66

Went and picked up the boys. Told my oldest what the Dr. said, and he teared up. He told me he had a dream 2 years ago that I was in a casket. He woke up crying and went to his dad and step mom. Breaks my heart that this could be a reality soon.

February 14, 2015

11:30pm 101/59 HR 60

Super tired this morning. Had 2 clients, then got ready for my date with the boys. Took them to Red Robin then to the Silvertips game. Had so much fun with them. Told my middle son about what the Dr. said today, and I don't think he understands it like my oldest does. I just want to spend as much time with them as I possibly can doing fun things. I'm worried that it won't be much longer before I'm not gonna have the energy to do much. But on a good note, this was one of the best Valentine's days ever.

February 15, 2015:

10:48am 97/53 HR 55

4:31pm 116/65 HR 80

9:05pm 98/59 HR 80

Had a very relaxing day. Boys spent a good portion of today outside playing, it was such a beautiful day. So nice having them for 3 nights. My youngest, later on tonight, wasn't feeling too well. He came and laid in bed with me and fell asleep. I hope he isn't sick. My middle son has been complaining of a sore throat for a couple days. Been giving him silverbiotics and day/nightquil to see if he feels better.

I just hope I don't get sick. I'm really scared if I do. I don't want to end up in the hospital again.

February 16, 2015:
9:26am 88/52 HR 73
10:01am 102/61 HR 73
Super dizzy and exhausted today. Ran out of fludro yesterday. Waiting for the Dr. to refill it at the pharmacy.
2:33pm 99/60 HR 80
Took about a 30 min nap after cleaning the house. Super exhausted today. Hopefully I can sleep good.
10:20p, 95/56 HR 80

February 17, 2015:
10:26am 88/52 HR 55
Super exhausted. Took a nap and then went to craft night for a friends Bday party.

February 18, 2015:
I have been awake since 3:30am. It's gonna be a very long day.
Started my BC yesterday. Hopefully it will help with the acne.
11:12am 98/61 HR 81
Nice to have some time to myself today. Music therapy, dancing and just enjoying me time.
2:10pm 94/60 HR 72

February 19, 2015:
9:19am 111/60 HR 79
Fell asleep about 9pm last night. Woke up about 8 times, but fell quickly back asleep, slept til 8:30am. Feel a bit rested, but also like I could still sleep.
8:45pm 102/61 HR 79

Took about a 15 min nap today, but was able to lay and rest for 90 min. House was such a mess when I got home. Only took me 10-15 min to clean it, but no one else can bother, because video games are more important? I can't stress how much I've said no games for my youngest after school, yet every time my brothers watch him, he is playing when I get home from work. Kind of glad I have a short day tomorrow. I need to get some me time.

February 20, 2015:
Slept crappy last night, super tired today.
1:02pm 112/73 HR 80
Took an hour nap while my youngest was at school.
10:08pm 110/77 HR 68

February 21, 2015:
9:48pm 99/61 HR 73
Had a full day at the office. Which was really nice.
Went to my friends F.R.I.E.N.D.S themed party. So fun to hang out and eat.
Poked myself really hard in the eye. Instant headache and I felt pain for like 5 min in the back of my head.
Feeling super exhausted tonight. Took some melatonin, hoping to get some good sleep.

February 22, 2015:
Slept so good last night
9:23am 104/60 HR 81
4:23pm 98/60 HR 80
Still haven't heard from the Dr. about my 24-hour heart monitor. I don't want to call and ask for it, but I know I have too. I really should switch my Drs. I'm not fond of him, but once this other insurance kicks in and I get more answers I can.

I hate the chest pain that I have, especially when it stops me in my tracks. I just want everything to be level now. I hate waiting and testing and changing every month.

Good news is my oldest brother will be out in 7 days. That will be a huge stress relief for me.

Got to spend some time to myself today which was so nice.

9:25pm 114/60 HR 80

February 23, 2015:

Didn't sleep again last night. Got up and took my middle brother to the bus stop, then went and dropped off a friend at the airport. Tried to nap but just couldn't fall asleep.

2:20pm 99/70HR 79

6 more days and it will all be done. Praying these days fly by fast.

February 25, 2015:

Had a fun night. Picked up a friend (who I hadn't seen for a long time) from the airport and hung out. So much fun.

4:25pm 99/60 HR 71

Took a nap today, still feeling groggy and unmotivated, but I really want to make a good dinner tonight.

Took BP after 20 min hot bath-7:19pm 1052/55 HR 92

February 27, 2015:

10:06am 100/67 HR 71

This morning I'm getting the 24-hour heart monitor put on. Not looking forward to it, but the past few days have been pretty hard on my heart, so I guess it's a good thing. At least I'll have the boys today through the weekend.

I'm so happy my oldest brother is leaving on Monday. Such a big relief.

1:48pm 99/67 HR 72

March 1, 2015:

10:36pm 102/65 HR 79

Wearing the heart monitor for 24 hours was so irritating. Glad it was only for 1 day. I didn't have to work or do much. But last night in bed, would have been a great read for it.

I didn't sleep well either. I guess after 2 good sleeps, my body was like, ok that's good.

March 2, 2015:

5:50pm 96/69 HR 69

Yay!! My oldest brother is moved out. WHOOHOO!!!! Now I just have a lot of cleaning to do in my middle son's room, since my middle brother moved into the open room. Once we have our house back, I will start on my Audrey Hepburn themed walk-in closet/bedroom. It will be nice to be back to just us.

Making some changes at my office, which I'm pretty excited about. Just have to plan it out.

10:20pm 107/52 HR 60

I feel like my BP is everywhere. No steady reading especially with the bottom number. My pulse is all over the place as well. But I am glad I noticed that when my body starts to relax-that is when my heart has all the issues, and when I'm really relaxed-that is when it's at its worst.

It's been nice having the few good days in a row. I really hope that it stays this way.

I've been getting up around 8-8:30am with energy and keeping it all day. I feel it helps with my busy Thursday's. Those are the hardest days. I feel like I use all my "spoons."

Praying everything goes well and I just start feeling more like myself. I really need to do more things for myself-even when I think it's selfish, because if I don't, I might go insane.

Really wanted to workout tonight with my husband, but he got home way too late. I don't feel tired tonight, but I will be taking Benadryl and melatonin to help with that.

The past couple days I've had period type cramps. Really annoying. I know it's only been 2 weeks on the BC, but I feel it's making me break out even more. Sucks, but I'll give it 2 months (or 2 pill packs) then I might just try *Yaz*, even though it hasn't had the greatest reviews.

March 4, 2015:

11:07am 107/67 HR 81

Last night I had horrible cramps. It was so painful.

2:42pm 105/68 HR 79

Today has been rough. Went and got the flooring for the waiting area.

Having a hard time with chest tightness and breathing.

Extremely fatigued today. I hate these days so much. It's not fair.

March 8, 2015:

1:25pm 126/70 HR 90

Allergies are really kicking me and my youngest son's ass again. Taking Benadryl is so hard on me because it just knocks me out. Gonna have to take me, my youngest, and oldest son in for allergy shots soon. I want to be on top of it this year. I feel like a zombie.

I also have been having bad cramping and spotting for about 5 days now. Super annoying.

March 11, 2015:

9:49am 103/59 HR 107

I have been spotting since March 3rd. So tired of all this. Just stop already.

Last 2 days I've had 0 energy.

Today I feel better, minus the horrible cramps.

March 12, 2015:

8:57pm 108/63 HR 72

Felt sick all day. No longer just feeling like allergies. I feel like I'm running a fever, slight body chills.

My BP is good, so I need to keep monitoring that, so it stays up. Want to be on top of stress dosing if I need to.

Such a long day at the office. There from 930am-815pm.

I need to sleep amazing tonight.

March 13, 2015:

10:33am 90/52 HR 64

11:49am 88/56 HR 60

2:22pm 100/58 HR 71

Resting in bed all day. So sick, dizzy, weak, sore throat, chills, and fast potties. UGH! This is horrible. Stuffy nose, headache. Just want this to be over.

4:19pm 98/56 HR 74

6:22pm 112/67 HR 89

8:22pm 98/54 HR 68

11:13pm 80/51 HR 65

11:22pm 95/42 HR 64

March 14, 2015:

9:12am 93/51 HR 60

9:54am 96/61 HR 65

11:06am 97/61 HR 67

1:50pm 99/56 HR 73

2:45pm 97/59 HR 69

I hate being in bed. I hate being sick. This sucks! It was nice having my friend visit today and she brought me juice (mean green) to help with the cold.

My middle brother got his 2 checks from school today. So hopefully he will start looking for a place to be out by this weekend. Would be great to have the house back. Him and my husband cleaned up the porch and backyard, which was a huge help.

6:16pm 114/65 HR 74

7:48pm 98/64 HR 60

10:34pm 98/64 HR 81

If I'm not better by tomorrow I am going to have to go to the walk-in or ER. Not sure what they can do, but I have to get better soon.

March 15, 2015:

9:20am 88/66 HR 72

9:40am 98/63 HR 55

11:01am 97/52 HR 60

11:46am 88/53

Went to the ER today. I felt so off and just couldn't pull myself out of it. I was really scared that something bad might happen and I am still not exactly sure what an adrenal crisis really is. I have only had one and I don't know if it will be the same thing each time (I am sure it's different all the time, because this doesn't feel exactly like the first one). With my BP being off all day, I didn't want to take any chances. I was feeling extremely lethargic and to be honest, I was really scared. I was being to prideful and wanted to convince myself that I had it under control. I know it's just a cold, but I also don't want to put myself in any danger of slipping into a coma or dying, so I put my pride aside and had my husband take me in. When we got to the ER they gave me 3 bags of fluid and some HC, just to be on the safe side. My BP was steady at 107/75 with HR in the 60s. With my vitals back to normal, they let me go home. Still feeling horrible, weak, dizzy, and exhausted. Ready for this day to be done.

March 17, 2015:

Woke up feeling about 80% better. I have some energy today, but don't want to overdo it. I am gonna get dressed and make myself look presentable since I've looked like I should live under a bridge the last 5 days.

March 18, 2015:

Fell asleep around 11pm, woke up and looked at my phone, said it was 2:30am. Fell back asleep, woke up again, looked at my phone, said it was 1:20am. Got really confused, was then up til 2:30am before I finally fell back asleep. Thought I heard my youngest crying, so I got up, at this point it's 3:30am. Wasn't him, it was a cat either dying or giving birth. Haven't been able to fall back asleep. Ugh!! Bring on the day......

Dr. Results: Heart thingy came back, nothing to be too concerned about and it's looking ok. I just need to lower my stress to reduce the palpitations and get them regular. Upped my meds..... AGAIN. UGH!! Go back in 2 weeks for blood draw to check all my levels.

I need to get my allergies under control so that it is not stressing my body out, I need to not take on so much and slow down a bit. Learn to use my energy wisely. BLAH BLAH BLAH........

March 23, 2015:

Spent the weekend with my best friend/sister. We had such a fun time. Talking and hanging out. I love her so much. Seeing her makes me miss home. I want to move back to Eastern Washington. I really hate Western Washington.

Had to take my youngest to the ER yesterday. My husband's shin Landed on my youngest sons Achilles. Did not slow him down though. But after being home for a bit he said it felt like it was beating like his heart. He is not putting all his pressure on it and says when he walks on his toes it hurts less. It is pretty swollen though. Nothing stops this child from moving at 100mph.

March 28, 2015:

Bit it hard core in the kitchen tonight. The floor was wet, and I went down hard. Sat and iced my leg and hip. I feel like my body is 100 years old.

April 3, 2015:

My middle brother moved out a couple days ago and I got to make the extra room my Audrey Hepburn themed walk-in closet. I painted the walls Tiffany blue with black and pink trim. Drew a pic of her eyes and lips on one of the walls. Painted a couple of her quotes on my furniture. It's so beautiful. I love coming here and sitting on my huge movie sac (if you don't know what that is, go visit a Lovesac store. They are so amazing and comfortable).

So nice having everyone out and it just being us again.

I also got 3 other rooms organized and cleaned. Spring cleaning sucks but getting rid of extra stuff feels amazing. 4 more rooms to go.

OMG I am still in pain from doing the room set up and cleaning everything. It was too much for my body to handle but it looks so amazing.

April 24, 2015:

Waiting to get my blood drawn. I hate doing this. I feel like they take way more than they need. It always makes me feel dizzy. I know that I need to have it done to check all my levels, but I wish there was an easier (and faster) way.

May 7, 2015:

Got my blood results back...UGH!!!! Thyroid and kidney levels are good so that's a plus. Cortisol levels look good, so I am on the right dosage for that finally. Potassium levels are really low, Renin levels are suppressed (????) and I'm still apparently "pre-diabetic." I have to wait til the 27th to find out what the heck this all means. Why do they have to wait so long? I get that if it was an emergency, they would get me in sooner to talk about it, or at least I hope they would, but the waiting game sucks and it's stressful.

May 22, 2015:

My body and joints are in a lot of pain today. I feel like I am always over doing it, but I also feel like I hardly do anything. I really hate this disease.

May 27, 2015:

Another med adjustment and blood drawn....

Because of the shirt I wore into the Dr. today, he advised me that if I drink beer, then I need to be eating salty things with it to balance it all out. I did get to tell him that I don't drink beer, I just get to wear the shirts thanks to Trivia nights.

Walking into our bedroom, I almost stepped on a tarantula. OMG talk about heart attack. I think burning the house down is a good idea. Talk about sending me into an adrenal crisis. THEY ALL MUST DIE!!!

May 28, 2015:

Zero energy. Needing the hubby home to take care of our youngest and bring me meds.

I hate getting sick.

May 30, 2015:

Finally getting to rest. Hoping to feel better by tomorrow. Colds really take a toll on your body when you have a shitty immune system. Seems like having a cold with Addisons is 10x worse than when I had them when I was healthy.

May 31, 2015:

Lying in bed, sick, watching *Ever After*. One of my favorites to watch when I am not feeling well. For some reason it helps me feel better.

June 1, 2015:

This stupid cold has taken a toll on my body. I want to get back to working out, but I barely have energy to get dressed. Time to push myself, but I know that if I do that, it will only make things worse. Praying this cold ends soon, so I can get back into my routine.

June 6, 2015:

Went wine tasting with friends. It was so much fun going to all the different wineries, sampling new things and just having some girl time.

It did take all my energy to make it through, and it was painful, but I am glad that I was able to do something fun after being sick for so long.

June 8, 2015:

Missed 2 weeks of working out due to being sick and recovering… Back at it this morning. Easier to get back in it this time. Feeling good. Just got to keep myself healthy and away from all the germs out there.

June 14, 2015:

My friend threw me an amazing Audrey Hepburn themed birthday party. So many people came out, dressed up, drank, and had fun. This has been the best birthday yet. I love themed parties.

My feet felt like they were going to fall off, but I had a ton of fun. I know that I will be paying for it the next couple days, but I can't stop having fun because of it.

June 22, 2015:

Hate having these stupid chest heaviness episodes. They went away for a while, but now they are back. UGH!!! Just breathe and try not to think about it. It seems to just happen when I am resting. Like my body starts to stress too much when I am relaxing, which is weird.

July 1, 2015:

Major headache, sore throat, body chills, joint pain, zero energy... I have shit to do today, why does this happen to me. I was just sick, why am I sick again???

July 2, 2015:

Still feeling crappy. I hate being this sick. I feel worse than I did yesterday. The dizziness and nausea are horrible today. I feel like my body is trying to kill me.

Had to swallow my pride and let my husband take me to the ER.... I hate this place. They know nothing about Addisons and always try to just give me pain meds. Yes, I am in pain, but it's not like the pain meds kind of pain. I can't seem to explain it to people in a way they would understand because they don't go through this kind of pain. I can't take pain meds, because they make me really sick, and with how I am already feeling, I don't think the added symptoms would be something my body could handle. Really low BP when I first got here, but after a few bags of saline and some HC, my vitals got back up to a normal level. I really hope the extra fluids will help me kick this adrenal crisis in the ass and help with this "cold" like illness going on in my body. I hate feeling so out of it. I could barely form words when I first got there, it was extreme brain fog.

Home and resting now. I don't want to be sick for the 4th of July. I want to be able to enjoy it with my friends. Why did this happen to me???

July 3, 2015:

Extra doses of Hydrocortisone sure helped. Feeling better today, just really weak.

I love getting to clean the pots that have been sitting on the stove since Tuesday. The smell was fantastic. Good thing I started feeling better, the house was looking pretty nasty. I shouldn't be the only one doing things. Shit needs to still get done when I am sick, so I don't have to do everything when I am still recovering.

July 6, 2015:

This stupid cough really needs to go away. Plus, I need some energy. Stress dosing might come in handy til this cough goes away.

July 9, 2015:

Not quite 100% myself but getting there. This cough has got to go though. I swear it's just hanging on to annoy me.

July 17, 2015:

So happy we got to actually spend a day doing fun things with the kids today. The boys are so excited.

Thank God I am finally feeling better and had the energy to get out and do something.

July 22, 2015:

Got our allergy test results back. I'm sensitive to wheat but not gluten…… Surprised that my oldest is more sensitive to gluten then my youngest. We are all sensitive to eggs, (especially my youngest) soybean, corn, and casein.

This diet change should be fun.... But hopefully it will help with some of my symptoms.

July 26, 2015:

Spent the weekend with my best friend/sister and another amazing friend. Was able to relax by the pool. Took a nap. Went bar hopping in Wenatchee. I was in a lot of pain but held it together pretty well. We went and saw *Train* at the *Gorge*. First time I had ever been there, and it was so beautiful. The weekend festivities really took me out though. It was rough.

August 16, 2015:

So much fun this weekend. Loved having time with my boys, had a blast at *Silverwood*. Got to spend time with my best friend/sister and my adorable nephews. Glad to be out of the car!!!!
So much driving. My body did not like that at all. Overall my body held up pretty good. I felt that I had enough energy to make it through that day.

August 19, 2015:

Woke up to my youngest screaming/crying at 2:30am. I take 2 steps out of our bedroom and see why. Big, huge, ginormous spider in front of the bathroom door. You know it's big when you can see it from that far away. I scream for my husband to come kill it. He was even scared, but he killed it. I now have a fear that there are more, and they will kill us because we killed its leader. If we owned the house I would suggest burning it down and starting over. Time to get crazy with some spider killer. I think 100 gallons should cover it.

August 21, 2015:

Still trying to recover from last weekend and missing 3 doses in 8 days. I keep pushing myself and today I was really feeling it.

I have too much to get done this weekend, so body, if you could please cooperate and let me have the energy and pain free weekend that would be great.

I managed to push through and it felt like it was an out of body experience, minus the actual pain that I did feel the whole time. Why does my back have to cause so many issues.... All the time.

August 30, 2015:

I've been horrible this weekend and ate and drank about everything I'm not supposed to have.... And I'm feeling it. Time to get back on track, because how it all made me feel is not something I want to experience again.

September 7, 2015:

Stupid pharmacy has been closed since Friday. Been out of 1 of my meds since then and they don't open til tomorrow. I am really feeling it today, zero energy. I can't keep letting this happen. I have to be on top of keeping my meds filled, because missing days can really do a number on me.

September 8, 2015:

Ok body and mind...I really could use some sleep...Been trying to fall asleep since 9pm... It's 2am now.

September 13, 2015:

Having so much fun camping. Our youngest boy is doing amazing, he loves the outdoors. I am feeling pretty good. Back pain sucks, but I feel that I am not having any Addisonians moments.... yet.

September 28, 2015:

So happy I see my endocrinologist Wednesday. I need a med adjustment so bad, because I have been overly exhausted, and can barely make it through all the days, along with other weird symptoms. I HATE this, but it's my life now, and it's all about making adjustments.

September 29, 2015:

I don't think I actually slept last night. I was in a constant in-between state. Today is gonna be rough.

As rough as it was, I did make it through. Sometimes I wonder how I get shit done feeling like this, but at least I get shit done.

September 30, 2015:

If you are a young nurse.... DO NOT talk to your patients like they are children. I am old enough to take care of my own shit. I don't want to come to see my Dr. and be treated like a child. No, it's not being polite. I am an adult, more so than you... So Please address me as such. 20-year-old's annoy me more than ever.

What do you do when your Dr. says "don't work so much," but you have an interview, so you can work more?...... Nail that interview and see where life takes you. Wish me luck!

Got the job at my favorite Spa.... I will be at the spa a few nights a week and I am still going to keep my business, so no changes there.

October 7, 2015:

Wow. 1 year ago, I was diagnosed with Addisons. Still trying to get my meds figured out. Still trying to get this life figured out and how to pace myself. I think that if I can still push myself to do what I want until my body says STOP, I will do that.

October 16, 2015:

Can't wait to crawl into my bed. My body has had enough of today. I have over used it and it's not happy. I don't want to speak this into my life, but I feel like I am starting to get sick.…. Again.

October 21, 2015:

Woke up with a sore throat and stuffed nose.... Tea tree oil, Flonase, and silverbiotics are my best friends today. I honestly feel like I was just sick.…. Is this going to happen every month?

October 23, 2015:

This stupid cold has knocked me down. Resting again today. I hate being sick, especially when the house is a mess.

October 25, 2015:

Over did it yesterday, now I feel worse and have zero energy. Why can't I just learn to rest when I am sick?… Oh ya, because I am the only one who can apparently get anything done around the house.

October 26, 2015:

This cold is really kicking my ass.

October 31, 2015:

Went and got the rest of my Halloween costume. Me, my husband, and our friends dressed up as the cast from *Arrow*. I always love getting dressed up. Took the kids out trick or treating. My body did not like all that walking around in the cold.

When we got home, I noticed my youngest kept scratching his head. I decided to just look to see what he was scratching at. I hardly moved his hair and saw that he was infested (yes, infested, you could see them moving around without moving his hair) with head lice. I was mortified. We just had all of our friends over with their kids… Those calls were fun. Thankfully all our friends are amazing and understanding.

Had to shave him completely bald because they were not coming off. Good thing he is a boy. He hates his hair (or lack thereof) right now, but he will get over it.

November 15, 2015:

Just saw that I missed my meds Friday night, both am and pm on Saturday, and today's morning meds. No wonder I have felt so drained and feel like I can barely function today. This is not good. I really need to set an alarm or something, so I can remember to take them.

November 21, 2015:

Full day of cleaning and getting the house back to normal, then a full schedule at the spa. I'm so exhausted, but my brain says, let's stay up and ponder life. Will I ever get good sleep again? Or is this going to be my life? My no sleep life.

December 15, 2015:

Got the boys bunk bed all pulled out and ready to assemble. The first thing I noticed was the railing for both sides for the top was bent. Not a big deal, but still not happy with that. Had to hammer some parts to get them to match up with where the screws went. Going along and realized, they didn't give us any of the plastic plugs or slat spacers for the top. So, missing a bag of important pieces, big deal. I'm putting the metal slats on and we have 15.... You need 22. So those are missing. I keep assembling while I am on the phone with the company. After I call, they say, "call back a little later," they are fixing their phone lines. Get to the futon part of the bed......
MISSING ALL THE PIECES on the 2nd page of the parts page. So, I call again... On hold for 24 min.... oh they don't make the metal ones, they only make the wood ones, so they give me the number for the right place....
Been on hold for 20 min. GREAT DAY!!!!
Talk about trying to avoid stress… How do you avoid shit like this??

December 17, 2015:

Some parents are just ignorant and hateful. UGH. I don't have to explain why my son is how he is to everyone who wants to comment on his behavior. Keep your comments to yourself. He is an amazing boy with so much love.
I get that some kids are brats and annoying, which my son is not. There is obviously something that isn't "right" with him. Plus, he is 7 years old... He's supposed to be "spastic" and crazy. He's a boy. I would like to punch those parents in the face… Again, how do I avoid stressful situations like this?

December 26, 2015:

Ugh... Still trying to figure out meds. Will I ever get this down? I am so glad that I will be seeing a new endocrinologist in January. Hoping for a better new year.

December 31, 2015:

Little bit of a traumatic night, but we are home safe. My oldest was zoning out while driving and came razor close to hitting a guard rail. I have a horrible headache, blurry vison, shakiness, and still trying to come down from the "incident."

I am wanting/needing to go to bed, but the boys are so wired and loud.

******

This time in my life was horrible. I honestly don't know how I did it. It was almost like it was a very depressing/scary dream. My marriage was still struggling, and I was pushing those issues aside. Letting the stress of it eat at me. I was still able to make it to a lot of the boy's games, but the stress of traveling was really tearing up my body. My back was still in a ton of pain and I was just trying to ignore it all. Both my brothers were living with us and I hated being home in the chaos and mess. I was not listening to the rest, I think, that my body was craving. I was battling depression that I was obviously ignoring and I was letting my life fall apart but acting like I had all my shit together. Inside, I was screaming for help and my disease was taking over and thriving. I still wasn't taking the disease seriously, yet I was researching it all the time. To me, I was still able to do things, not like I used to, but I was still working and having some sort of a life. I didn't look sick, but I sure felt it. I put on a good act around everyone. I didn't want anyone to know I was scared and falling apart.

SICK WIFE

On top of being a sick mom, I have to be a sick wife. I feel this is more challenging. The stress of being married when you are healthy is bad enough, but when you add your sickness to it, that becomes a real issue.

I have read so many posts on social media, where the spouse will leave because the stress of having to take care of their sick spouse has gotten to be too much for them. I get it, it's a lot. I am not sure I could handle it, but I am in the opposite situation, I am the sick spouse. At any moment my husband can decide to leave me because he doesn't want the burden, stress, and distance this "diseased" relationship has now caused.

My husband is 9 years younger than me. He doesn't have any biological children, but my youngest son, whom he adopted, is his son. I know that he wanted to have a biological child, but I am not willing to have a child in my condition. I know people with Addison's have babies all the time. People with Fibromyalgia have babies all time. Women in their late 30's have babies all the time. I do not want to try and raise a baby when I am this sick. When I have a hard enough time taking care of my own children. I am so thankful they are old enough to fend for themselves. I am thankful that my oldest, who is now an "adult" and can take care of himself.

I am thankful I got to do all the hard parts when I was healthy. It might sound selfish, but I couldn't give a new born what it needed. I feel I would resent my husband for making me have another baby. I would be the one who would have to care for it... No, My boys would be the ones who would have to care for it mostly. Most days they have to care for me. It would not be fair.

I know my husband wants to travel, go on dates, go to concerts, be young and have fun. I can't do those things for two reasons: 1: I am in my late 30's, so going out to bars and that kind of stuff isn't appealing to me anymore. 2: I am to sick most of the time, too worried about being around people, and too stressed just thinking about it.

I often feel that this is not fair to him. I feel like I am robbing him of having a great, fun, and exciting relationship with someone new. I feel like I am robbing him of having a biological child of his own. The stress of this relationship on me and trying to be a good mom and not having time or energy to put into being a good wife… That is not fair to him.
He is a good guy. He wants to take care of me. He wants to spend his life with me. But in my mind, how long will those "wants" of his change to "cant's?"

I am not scared to be alone. I am not scared that he will leave. He and I would be friends and I know he would help me out in every way possible to make sure that I was taken care of. I know he would be over all the time checking on me, seeing if he could help with anything, and making sure the boys saw him. He would be the perfect ex. I don't want to hold him back from a life that he could be happy in.

We do go to therapy and talk about it all. He feels that I am ready to get out of this relationship. He feels that I am pushing him away. In a sense, he is right. I want him to be happy. I don't want him to think that I am only staying in it to have someone take care of me since I don't work.

This is so hard. Being a healthy wife was so much easier. We did so much together and had a great time. Even when I was first diagnosed we were fine and still did things. Then the fibromyalgia came on and it took such a toll on my body, because I refused to rest and pushed myself past my limits all the time. I feel I made myself sicker; faster. Now we can't even go on dates. We haven't had sex in 8 months. We haven't kissed in about 7 months. We haven't even touched, cuddled, or hugged in 8 months. I don't have the energy. Sex hurts. Being touched hurts. He works from 2:30pm-11pm, so that doesn't leave us time to be "intimate." I am so exhausted by 7pm, I can barely get my son in bed. I just don't have the energy. On his days off, he likes to spend as much time as possible with the boys, cleaning the house, getting errands done. By night time, we are exhausted. I know he would love to have sex, but the thought of it, stresses me out. Will it hurt me for days? Will it just be awkward and unenjoyable?

It's hard. I feel sorry for him. I feel sorry for me. We are trying to make this work, it's just a matter of time before we figure out which way we will eventually have to take. Whether we get divorced or stay together, I know that he will be here for me.

FIBRO MOM

I had all these new fun symptoms that came on, and just like always, I ignored them. It got to the point where I just couldn't any more. So, in January 2016, I went to my Naturopath and told her every weird thing that was happening in my body. She said it sounded like Fibromyalgia. Great! Another fucking disease. She had me go to my Endo for a second opinion. I went in on January 19th. Yep. She agreed. She ran some tests to make sure it wasn't arthritis. Fibromyalgia it is. This was killing me. I had a couple clients who had Fibro, but I wasn't really sure what it was and what it could do to you, so I went and researched it. That is all I needed on top of chronic back pain and Addison disease.

Journal Entry: January 2016- February 2016

January 10, 2016
Got my hair done. Needed a change and got some bangs.
I've been doing lots of traveling for the boy's games. It has been so stressful on my body I can't seem to recover from all the traveling.
Struggling this year with getting my youngest off to school after break. He cries and throws a fit when it's time to go to school. Breaks my heart to see him act like that.
Printer broke so had to go to Office Depot to get a new one. Can this year get better already?

January 13, 2016
When it's too painful to sleep: bed heater turned up, Audrey Hepburn movie on.... Hopefully sleep will over power the pain.

Did not sleep good at all, but I still have to try to function today. Finally, an Endocrinologist who knows what is going on... Lots of bloodwork, but should have results soon.... I love her. She actually knows what she is talking about and told me how serious I need to take this disease. It's not going to be an easy road, but she has been more helpful in this one visit then my other Dr. was in all of his combined.

January 19, 2016

Addisons.... Fibromyalgia.... bring it on. Just another excuse to run, get massages, and appreciate life.
I can't believe I have another autoimmune. I knew that there was a chance of one coming on at some point, I just didn't think it would be this soon. I have been trying to ignore some of the symptoms, and I have to stop doing that, but this explains why I always feel so shitty.

January 26, 2016

My body feels like there is an electric current running through it... I'm sure if I concentrated hard enough, I could shoot lightning bolts through my hands. Pain, pain, go away. I need sleep... and less stress in my life.

February 10, 2016

Apparently, I've ran 81.7 miles this year already. Not too bad, but gotta step it up... if my body will cooperate. I have been too hard on my body. My legs are still swollen from last night, and very tender. Walking is so painful right now.

February 28, 2016

Feeling the sickness trying to creep in.... But I'm not gonna let it take over. I swear, my body waits til it's over one cold, just to catch another one.
I decided to quit working at the spa. It was becoming too much on my body and having to work late nights was killing me. I felt like I just kept getting sick from being around everyone and their germs. I love working there, but I have to listen to my body.

******

My husband and I separated in March 2016, I was not happy. We were just making each other miserable, we would fight constantly, and he never helped me around the house. I was always mad at him. It wasn't just him; it was dealing with the pain and diseases too.

My husband didn't understand what I was going through, so he just pulled away and I pushed him away as well. I couldn't take being around him anymore. Every time I saw him, it would just anger me and stress me out. I needed him gone. If he didn't care to help, then he could leave.

He went and stayed with his mom. With him gone, I had to get a job, on top of running my own massage business. I had moved my business to my house, so it was easier on me. I got a job at a chiropractic office in April and was working while my youngest was at school, and then I would take on my own clients at home. My work week looked like this: Monday-Friday was 9am-8pm and a few clients on the weekends. I was able to move my home clients around, so I didn't have to miss a lot of the boy's games. My husband would take my youngest on his weekends off or when he would get off work early. I didn't realize what kind of abuse I was about to put my body through and what it would cost me.

Journal Entry: March 2016- September 2016

March 9, 2016

Woke up with a sore throat and my legs were swollen. It was painful to walk, but once I got moving around it got better. Glad I'm getting a massage today.

Thankful I'm getting my allergy shots today. Maybe this will help with giving my body a rest from attacking itself all the time.

Feeling weak, tired, and exhausted. Throat is swollen and sore... I will not get sick, I will not get sick... Ya, I am sick.

March 10, 2016
Being sick sucks and today I feel horrible, but I am so lucky that my husband decided to help out while I'm not feeling well. He got the kitchen cleaned, wood brought in, living room picked up, and gave me the bed to have all to myself, so I can rest. Lucky, lucky me...... I wish this happened all the time, but this is really the first time he has done this. I will praise him for it and maybe, it is something he will continue to do...

March 20, 2016
Talked to a friend about how I was feeling about my husband and I decided that it was time for us to separate for a while. It has been such a hard time for us for so long and it seems we just keep drifting apart. I can't keep that stress in my life. I am hoping the separation will help us figure out what to do.

March 27, 2016
Almost 2 hours of lawn mowing=zero energy today.
My husband is looking for a place to move into. We just fight so much now and can't stand to be around each other. My stress level has elevated, and it's been a struggle health wise. I should be stress dosing through this.
I have to start looking for a job, so I can support me and the boys. It's the last thing the Drs. want me doing, but I can't survive on what I am making with my business.

March 28, 2016
I do work and it exhausts me, but this won't define me or keep me from doing what I love. Massage is something I am good at and I don't want to have it taken away because of this disease. I will not allow it.

April 3, 2016

About 90 min of mowing. Which means I'll have zero energy for 2 days, and I start my week of 2 jobs tomorrow. Wish me luck.

April 20, 2016

Been nice having my husband out of the house. We seem to get along a little better and are talking like we haven't talked in a long time. My stress levels have gone way down with him gone. My body has had enough today though. Working 2 jobs might be the death of me.

April 25, 2016

Still have back issues. I feel surgery was the worst idea. It didn't help, and I think that it is what is causing the most stress on my body. If my back didn't hurt this bad, would the Addison's and Fibro bother me so much? I really need to get it taken care of, because it is almost debilitating most days.

April 26, 2016

Pain has been bad for about 4 days and the last 2 days have been horrible. I finally figured out why.... STOP eating foods you're sensitive to like it's a buffet. Time to detox and take my diet more seriously. I can't handle this pain. I know it's not just the diet. 2 jobs, single mom, stress of separation, and trying to make it to all the boys games... Yep, my life is a big stress ball of stress and pain.

May 1, 2016

My body hates me. Pushed it past it's point today and now I'm paying for it. Ugh
My husband and I are still talking and hashing things out, so this is good. I like that we can openly talk and get things out that we couldn't before.

May 5, 2016

My body has had enough of today. In bed resting, trying to gain energy for the weekend. If my body was only that simple. Like a battery that just needs to be recharged. But it is far from that and fails me almost daily.

May 29, 2016

Went home this weekend. Really needed that time away. I needed to be around my girls and to feel some peace. Going home always makes me feel better, it's a great reset. But again, my body didn't handle the traveling and I feel like I will be recovering for a few days.

June 2, 2016

Some days are harder than others... Today is that day. Fatigue has won, and I need to fight harder to get up and moving.

Craziest thing just happened. When I got home from work there was garbage all over the front yard. I went inside put some things away; grabbed a bag to go pick it up (maybe in the house for 5-7 min), walk outside.......
Gone. No one around. Am I losing my mind? I can't figure it out, but glad I didn't have to clean it up. So weird.

My husband and I have been getting along a lot better. Still have a TON to workout, but I like the communication that is going on. Some of it is in anger or resentment, or whatever you want to call it, but it is so nice to get it all out. We seem to get along during texts, but when we are actually with each other, it's a little awkward.

June 19, 2016

My husband and I got into it at my little birthday party. He started to yell at me in front of our friends. I was so embarrassed and pissed, I couldn't believe he would do that. I feel like this is never going to work. I can't have him stressing me out so much.

July 9, 2016

When your whole body is in pain and it even hurts to eat. Ugh. Why does this keep happening? Why can't I just have good days? I am so over these stupid diseases.

July 17, 2016

Got bit by something a few days ago and everyday it gets more painful, but it hasn't changed in size apparently. Can the pain just stop, this is ridiculous. It's a stupid spider bite and it has gotten to be so bad that I can't move my arm. I had a friend pop it. Now there is a big hole in my back. I hope it doesn't get infected, but at least I can move my arm. I can't believe one crawled into my bed and had the nerve to bite me. Little asshole.

July 24, 2016

Twisted my ankle today. Didn't think it was too bad, but it was painful. Now it's swollen more than I want it to be. I've got work and I have lots of stuff to do, so ankle, if you could please just stop hurting.... That would be great. Having to use the crutches, but they are just slowing me down.

July 28, 2016

When the hard decisions come, and you know you just have to move on. My husband and I are leaning more towards ending things maybe. I want him to date other people, and he found someone that he might be interested in at church so that is good. I want him to be happy and to be able to have what he wants. I just can't be that for him, but I am glad we are in a better place.

I do not want to date anyone. I just want to enjoy being single and focusing on my boys. Dating is way too stressful and I don't have time for that. My boys and my career are what I need to be focusing on.

The stress of all this is not something I want to take on right now.

July 31, 2016

Feeling so sick right now. Ugh. My stomach wants to throw up, but my brain is saying no. They need to work together and pick one.

August 14, 2016

That feeling when you snap your fingers and pain shoots all the way up your arm and into your neck... Good times.

August 16, 2016

After talking and figuring out how to make things work, my husband and I decided it would be best for us to put our youngest in private school. We are not happy with the changes the schools are making and parents not having any say and his IEP was a joke. He did his testing today and is pretty excited that he gets to go to school with his best friend.

August 27, 2016

My husband and I took our youngest to the fair. It was nice spending some time as a family and knowing we can get along as friends.

August 28, 2016

It's days like today that I really notice the severity of having Addison's and Fibro. How debilitating it can be, how hard I struggle just to get up to use the bathroom or get some water. Things still need to be done and I just can't do them, and I have to be ok with resting and helping my body try to gain some energy. So thankful my husband had our youngest today. Hoping I can recharge and make it through my day tomorrow. Saving up my spoons.

August 29, 2016

Should have taken another rest day. My body won't be able to handle much more if I keep pushing myself like this.

August 30, 2016

Ok body.... We just have to make it a few more hours. UGH

When you don't have that energy to make dinner, so you give your kid leftover rice.... he was not happy with me.

I have to be ok with resting and taking the time to heal so I can be here for my boys. If I keep pushing myself the way I have been I won't be here to see my boys grow into amazing men and I won't be here to see them have babies of their own. I need to start taking this seriously and know I can't be there for everyone and that it's ok to cancel things, so I can take care of myself. It's gonna be rough, but I've had too many scares the last couple weeks that have really opened my eyes. Being here for my kids is the most important thing and I need to save my spoons for them.

September 5, 2016

I have the best boys ever. Last night, my youngest got hurt and my middle son heard him crying, so he went and helped him. I didn't know til we got home, and he showed me the huge bruise on his leg and told me his brother helped him.

This morning, I'm doing the dishes and my oldest comes in and says, "I've got this mom ," and finished putting the dishes in the dishwasher for me. I am beyond blessed. They are my world and they make me so proud.

September 9, 2016

Insomnia sucks, pain sucks, nausea sucks, dizziness sucks, headaches suck.... pretty much my night. When you try to get comfortable but everything that touches you or you touch hurts. Trying to stay positive, but I just want a decent night's sleep, without pain, without nausea, and without dizziness. Just 1 night....

September 20, 2016

Yesterday marked our 6-year anniversary. We are working on fixing us, but I think it will be ok. We just need to keep communicating and being honest with each other. Maybe get into some couples therapy.

September 23, 2016

It feels like someone is tearing my muscles from my bones. Can I just have an hour of no pain.

September 26, 2016

My youngest has been sick the last couple days and now I am sick too. Can I please go 1 month without being sick.

September 29, 2016

Felt like my body was crushing itself last night. Hoping to get rest this morning. I need to be better tomorrow. Missing way too much work and life. I am afraid I am going to get fired because I can't make it in.
Still trying to figure out this stress dosing thing. Not easy. I am not sure how it works. I wish someone would explain it to me. I guess I could ask the Endo, but I don't want to look stupid.

September 30, 2016

I should listen to the Doctor. I've been pushing for so long now, my body hates me. I feel like it's deteriorating, and I can't stop it.

******

March to September I was doing ok. Still got sick a lot more than I should have (thanks shitty immune system). I could feel myself getting worn out, yet I continued to push myself past my limits. I was struggling health wise and the stress of massaging so much was taking a huge toll on my body.

My husband and I were getting along way better when we were apart. We talked a lot about how we were feeling and opening up about resentments and all the other mess of things we kept hidden from each other. We never did that when we were married. The boys were really upset about the separation, but they still got to see him a lot.

In October and November, I got really sick and couldn't kick it. I missed so much work, I was sure they were going to fire me. My body just didn't feel right and I couldn't get the energy to do anything. I missed out on the boy's games, I was in bed most of the time. Barely getting my youngest to school. I couldn't push myself any longer, I was fading fast.

Journal Entry: October 2016- November 2016

October 1, 2016
Was trying to throw my husband a "Prom" themed bday party (since he never got to go to his prom), but I have been so sick.
Everyone helped out and showed up. He was so surprised. I didn't last long and didn't help much because of being sick, but I am glad that he stayed and was able to have fun.
I went back home and crawled into bed while the boys helped take care of me.

October 2, 2016
100% sure my body is trying to kill me off right now. How long is this gonna hang on?

October 4, 2016
Sickness/pain/insomnia have won tonight.
Will this ever end. I always feel so dramatic, but FUCK!!!!

October 5, 2016
Starting to feel somewhat human again. Maybe I'll have enough energy to get dressed today.

Fibromyalgia added to Addisons disease is really killing me. It's like I can never heal.

My husband moved back in. It's a sink or swim type situation, so we shall see what happens.

October 9, 2016

My shoulders, up my neck and across my chest feels so achy, it's almost like they feel like they are burning. If I could just not have pain for 1 hour... That's all I am asking. Just one hour.

October 15, 2016

When you're in so much pain that your eyes keep watering.... Or is this crying?? Just need something to stop the pain right now.

October 25, 2016

Omg my body is hating me right now. Just need to fall asleep so I don't feel the pain. I don't understand how I can live like this. It's too much. I don't want to take pain meds and become addicted, but I can't totally understand why someone would. This fucking sucks.

October 27, 2016

I start my new meds today (low dose naltrexone). Hoping for results because today was not fun, pain wise. I'm tired of always being in so much pain. I'm tired of being so exhausted that it's hard to do something as simple as showering. I'm tired of not being able to do what I used to be able to do. Dr. says it will take about a month or 2 to see any change. I have been dealing with this for 2 years... What's 2 months?

October 28, 2016

When you are in so much pain, but you still have to make dinner for your son and carve pumpkins because he has been looking forward to it all week and you promised him. The struggle is real, but this mama has a fighter's spirit.

Instead of carving the pumpkins, I had him paint them. It was easier, and I didn't have to clean up a huge mess. He loved it.

October 30, 2016

The pain is so intense today. It feels like I am having contractions, but I am not pregnant. I spent most of the morning doubled over, it hurt too much to walk, and when I would move around the stomach pain intensified and I got super dizzy. I called my friend to ask her (since she is a nurse) what I should do and if it's something I can just wait out. She said to go in, but I want to see if resting in bed will help it go away…. Even though that's where I have been most of the day.

It's been a while, but the pain was too much tonight, and my pushy friend made me go to the ER. The nurse treated me like all I wanted was drugs. I kept telling her I can't have any because they make me sick, and then she said, "then what are you here for?" Fucking bitch, I'm here because I am in a lot of pain and want to know what is going on. She was awful.

Apparently low potassium can cause some very painful issues. Home and resting now.

November 5, 2016

Made it home from the Tri-Cities. Feel like it's gonna take a while to recover. This trip was a lot on my body.

Got really sick last night and I swear I threw up 2 days' worth of food. Scary night by myself in the hotel room. I went and walked around the mall with my son's team and grabbed some food to take back to the hotel. When I got back to the hotel, I ate my food and about 2 hours later I was throwing up and had the fast potties, blacked out for a moment, but made it back to the bed.

Felt a little better in the morning and was glad I was able to drag myself to see my oldest run at State Cross Country. Right now, I need the pain to dissipate and I need to be able to keep down some food… and my meds.

November 9, 2016

It's only the start of cold and flu season and I am sick for the 2nd time. Ugh. Hopefully it will pass quickly. I feel like death.

November 10, 2016
OK sickness, you can leave my body now. I don't have time for you to stick around. Time to stress dose.

November 12, 2016
I don't know what is going on with my head and vision, but it needs to get better. Today has not been great and it seems to be getting worse. Hopefully I can sleep it off. I love how I say, "sleep it off," like I actually get sleep.

November 15, 2016
I guess when you annoy a Dr. enough, they get you in asap lol. Got a call from the neurologist and they are squeezing me in tomorrow. I am nervous to see what might be causing these weird pains in my head. They have been going on for SOOO long, I don't know what I am expecting.

November 16, 2016
More meds. I have to keep a diary of symptoms and then go back in 6 weeks. If nothing has changed, they will do a CT or MRI. Ugh, I hate meds. He has me taking Topamax. He told me he believes they are cluster migraines... I do not think that is what they are. I have had several migraines, and this is nothing like that. He didn't really listen to what I was saying either.

November 17, 2016
Heading in, again, for more blood work for diabetes. I guess having Addisons means that I will forever be pre-diabetic. Not fun.
My shoulder, forearms, and stomach have been spasming like crazy today. On top of the pain, it's been a very exhausting day. Thanks to the pain getting worse as the day went on, I'm gonna have a fun time trying to fall asleep tonight.

November 22, 2016

I swear I get every sickness that goes around. Ugh. Can't catch a break. I've missed like a month of work already.

November 23, 2016

So tired of this dizziness. So tired of being sick and getting sick. This can't be the rest of my life.

November 24, 2017

Tonight, is one of those hard nights. Not to mention, almost having your hand broken because your husband still has night terrors. It's really annoying and he better get that shit figured out soon. I need my own room.

November 26, 2016

Definitely over did it the last couple of days, especially today. Would be nice to be able to have/hire help. The boys have been great though.

******

My husband and I decided that he could move back in and we would be more like roommates/dating. Trying to get to know each other again. I knew that this might either cause me more stress, or he would actually step up and realize how sick I really am and want to help make things a lot easier for me.

I wanted to change my diet up a bit, to see if that would help with how I felt. I decided to start juicing and that I would be do the vegetarian/seafood diet. I was feeling a bit better, but with how much I was working, it was just doing more damage than good.

Journal Entry: November 2016- April 2017

November 28, 2016

Day 8 of being sick with whatever this is. Can't seem to kick it out of my system. Started my juicing today. I sure hope it works. I'm so tired of daily pain. If I could just go back to the way it was with just having Addisons. That would be great! I was at least functioning and living then. I feel so dead right now. I want some sort of a life. Fibro has really taken the life out of me.

Had to smoke tonight because I haven't slept in almost 5 days. I need really good sleep. In bed at 7pm. YAY!

November 30, 2016

Day 2 of juicing. I have liked all the ones I've done. Now time to incorporate meals into it. I'll juice all day and eat dinner at night and slowly add in a meal in the afternoon in a few days. So far, I've had below 5 pain, which I don't know if it's because I got some sleep last night, or if it's from the juicing or the meds finally working.

I'm gonna continue with the juicing though. Really want to kick this cold. I'm so tired of being sick. I think the Topamax is giving me the insomnia too.

I don't know what is wrong with my husband, but he just stopped helping out a few weeks ago. Kinda right after he got his computer. All he wants to do is be on the stupid computer doing gaming stuff. He promised to read with my youngest every day, but that doesn't happen. I'm sick of it. He totally laid down when he got the letter from LNI about his hours. He has no fight in him, he just lets things be. Would be nice to see him fight for what he wants. Maybe it could work between us if he actually did that. I'm tired of him being a boy. I need him to be a man.

December 6, 2016

Sometimes life throws some hard punches and pushes you in a direction you didn't plan on. Sometimes it takes you away from something you love doing and forces you to focus on yourself. The choices I'm having to make because of my health are not what I am wanting to do, but what life has lead me to at this point. My body is not what it once was, and it is not going to get better if I don't listen to it. Right now, it's about being here for my kids as much as I can and putting the little energy I have into them. Pain, fatigue, and a whole lot of health issues have not won, just pushed me in another direction.

I hate having to give up massage, but my body just can't take the stress of it anymore. This breaks my heart.

December 8, 2016

Did 8 days of juicing and it helped. Didn't get to juice these last 2 days and I'm starting to feel it. I know keeping my body healthy with good foods in it is a must. My husband finally stepped back up and has been helping. It's so hard with him working so much and having to rely on him to help more. Very stressful on both of us. But he did get good news today, he will be starting at *Boeing* soon. Hopefully this will be really good for him.

I need to figure out my situation. I am not happy with the changes I have to make because of my health. I think it's making me depressed. I need to find a way to help out financially or I am going to lose it. I don't know why I can't just be ok with my husband making the money. I want my boys to see how hard I worked for what I wanted, and I know they do, but having to step back makes me feel so weak and vulnerable. I am not used to this and I hate it so much.

December 10, 2016

Just laid down in bed, and my low back feels like it's on the verge of spasming. Now I'm afraid to move positions. Why does my body hate me so much?

December 11, 2016

Starting to feel it creep up again. This time it's a sore throat. I hate cold/flu season. I was just sick, but every little virus finds its way to me. I guess that's what I get for having a shitty immune system.

December 13, 2016

Today was a lot on my body. My kitchen is a disaster because I had to decide what I needed to use my energy for. I wish I didn't have to choose, I want to be able to do it all.

December 15, 2016

Every step I take is so painful. Even driving is hard. If I cut off my legs, the pain won't be there anymore, right??? Would be nice to be able to take a step without it feeling like torture.

December 18, 2016

Still so painful to walk. This is so frustrating. It's worse than stepping on Legos.

December 19, 2016

The pain in my legs will go away today. I will be able to walk without it feeling like I'm being tortured. No more pain, no more pain……. If I just keep repeating this to myself, it will be. I wish it was that simple.

December 20, 2016

Great, my thyroid is now starting to show signs of an autoimmune disorder. Why thyroid? Why are you failing me now?
Gonna be making another diet change and trying a new med, but hopefully this will work for me. This past week has been hell. Having extreme pain when walking is awful, and I look like I'm 100 years old when I walk. Trying to hide the pain you are in is not easy.

December 24, 2016

Nursed my oldest all day yesterday and now it's hit me. Gotta try to keep everyone else from getting sick.
Juicing, day/nyquil, immune boosters, lots of water and rest. I will not let this sickness ruin our Christmas. We will all be better by tomorrow morning.

December 26, 2016
Pain is too much tonight. Makes it so hard to fall asleep.

December 28, 2016
Can this sickness please go away? I want a break, a nice long break.
Drove over to Eastern Washington to spend some time with my mom, but not sure I am going to be able to enjoy it when I feel so sick.

December 29, 2016
I'm over being sick. My nose is raw from blowing it so much. My body can't decide if it's cold or hot. The pressure from my sinuses feels like my head is giving birth... I'm done. So glad that I am at my mom's so she can take care of me.

December 30, 2016
We spent the weekend at my mom's. She helped take care of us while we were sick. It was nice to be pampered for once. My youngest threw up at mom's before we left and in the car on the way home. My sinus cold has now gained a cough. We are home and resting now.
It's never fun to travel when you are sick and worse when you have a sick child.

January 17, 2017
Drove 2½ hours in the crappy, crazy rain and wind, got home at 10:35pm, got my youngest in bed, cleaned the kitchen, picked up my husband from work, finished cleaning the kitchen, fed the girls, grabbed a quick bite to eat, got myself ready for bed...... pain level: 8.... Which means no sleep for me tonight. Over did it and I am sure it's going to come back and bite me in the ass.

January 19, 2017
1 year today with Fibromyalgia and in October it will be 3 years with Addisons disease, and now the possibility of other autoimmune diseases.

The past 6 months I've gone downhill but hoping it won't get worse. Gotta keep staying positive and learn how to take it easy and know my limits. I have amazing friends who are so understanding, and my boys have been so great. Time to get it all under control so I can have more good days and enjoy life.

January 23, 2017
Can barely get off the couch. This sickness needs to pass fast. I'm tired of getting sick every other week.

January 24, 2017
Feeling worse. Can't sleep. Nose is so congested, and my eyes keep watering. My whole body hurts.
The sinus pressure is a bit much. I want this sickness to be over already.... And not come back at least for a few months. My body really needs a break from being sick all the time.

January 26, 2017
One thing I love about Instagram is that it has connected me to others who struggle with autoimmune diseases. We can message each other, encourage each other, and see each other's struggles. It's been so nice to have that community.

January 27, 2017
Hurts so bad to swallow. No energy. I can see myself getting dehydrated, because trying to swallow water is torture.

January 28, 2017
Feeling about 60% better, cold wise, but I have no energy whatsoever. I took a 2-hour nap and feel like I could go to bed and sleep all night.

January 31, 2017

Made it home by 12:30am. 5 hours of driving, 4 hours of sitting in bleachers.... My body is not happy. So glad I can rest today. Watching the boys play ball, is worth the pain. Went to see my middle son play and thought I could catch the last quarter of my oldest son's game. When we showed up they were just warming up (didn't realize it was a boys and girls game) so I was able to watch his whole game as well.

The drive home was excruciating. I was in tears and just wanted to get home and make the pain stop.

Haven't been able to fall asleep because the pain is so bad. Now it's 6am and I haven't slept at all.

February 9, 2017

I hate being sick. I want to work so I can have money to see my boys more often. I always feel like I should just make the move down there and be close so me and my youngest can be with them. Not being able to work or make money is making it impossible. I can't do anything. I fear that I won't be around long, and I'll miss even more of their lives and they won't remember good times with me. Or they won't love me for not being there. Which I know is not true, they love me. They are the reason I breath and survive. I hope I can show that to them on a daily basis. I really need to get back into finishing my book. Wonder if I can make it as a writer one day?

February 28, 2017

Got more blood taken today to test for Lupus and see how my other levels are doing. She wants me to get tested for Lyme's disease and to check to see if mold could be a problem, and she's referring me to a rheumatologist for the fibro. She got on me for missing meds and not taking them earlier in the day as well.

Everything will come back normal and my health will get better!!!! Gotta stay positive because I really don't need another autoimmune disease. Talked to the rheumatologist's receptionist and she told me that they don't treat fibro, so there is really no point in making an appointment. Ok.... I guess that is one more thing I don't have to do. So, if a rheumatologist doesn't treat fibro, who does?? No one, because most Drs. think it's all in your head.

******

Starting in March my back got worse. It was to the point where there were days I couldn't walk at all. I thought all this time that it could be the Addisons and Fibro making it worse, but maybe it was the back pain that was making all my other symptoms worse. I decided it was time to make an appointment with my surgeon again and see what options we had. I also started seeing a therapist to try and face what I was feeling. I wasn't sure if it was going to help, but I knew I needed something.

My surgeon and I sat down and talked about everything going on and what we think would be the best options. I went home and thought about it and decided that I was so sick of being in this kind of pain. I thought the back pain was stressing my body out so much, that it was causing me to have more flares. I decided it was time to have the fusion. We got everything set up.

In June I started doing iron Infusions. Those did not go well. I had to go through 3 sessions. The first was the worst. An hour after, I felt so sick. I could barely move my arm where they had the IV placed. I was so tired, I couldn't function. That lasted for 3 days.

The next fusion went a little better. I still felt really sick and tired after, but I didn't have the arm pain. Same with the 3rd fusion. I had a few pre-op appointments (which I documented on my YouTube channel). Surgery was set for August 1st.

Journal Entry: March 2017-July 2017

March 1, 2017

Again with the horrific stomach pain. I feel like *Freddy Kruger* is trying to slice his way out of my stomach. Dizziness, nausea, vomiting from the pain. I just want it all to stop.

Today has been horrible and the pain just keeps getting worse. I don't know what to do.

I am at home with just my youngest and he has been checking on me. I keep telling him I am fine, but I know he knows that something is really wrong.

I am trying to hide the pain, but I just can't.

March 2, 2017

My youngest found me curled up on the bathroom floor at 2am. I was in and out of consciousness. He was going to call 911, but I told him to grab his dad. Little guy shouldn't have had to see his mommy in so much pain, but he was brave, and scared. He was the one pushing for my husband to take me in.

Again, I get a Dr. who knows nothing about Addisons disease and doesn't believe in Fibromyalgia. Thinking I am just another drug seeking addict. They ran a few blood tests, did an ultrasound, and gave me fluids and HC. The Dr. thinks it was a cyst on my ovary (since there was fluid in that area), but I don't think that caused the extreme stomach pain. It was mostly in my upper stomach and it made my ribs feel like they were giving birth to piranhas. The pain was so bad it had me throwing up and I could barely move. Every move felt like pure torture.

Home from the ER and feeling a bit better after the meds they gave me. Nauseous and dizzy, but it beats that horrific stomach pain I was feeling.

March 19, 2017

Got together with my sister/best friend and a couple other friends from home. We drank way too much. I honestly thought I was going to have to go to the ER yesterday. I was throwing up so much, I couldn't keep my meds down, or anything. I was dizzy, shaky, and had the sweats. My head felt like it was being pried open. The only thing that made it stop was smoking. So glad I bought some just in case I needed it... And I really did. I was able to function after smoking.

March 26, 2017
Well, I over did it today. Everything hurts, and I can barely walk now. When am I going to learn my lesson. I can't keep pushing my body til it can't even move.

March 27, 2017
Super shaky today. I am dropping things left and right. What is going on with the grip in my hands. Keeps getting worse.

March 31, 2017
Started seeing a therapist today. I hope that this will help with my depression. The first session went really well, I am so glad I finally decided to do this. I should have done this a long time ago. I didn't realize how bad things were until we got about half way through. I broke down and cried. I never cry, especially in front of strangers. I know this was a great first step in battling the depression that I like to pretend I don't have.
It's nice to know that she is understanding to the pain I am going through. Her in-laws have Lyme's disease, so she sees them going through a hard time and struggling to figure out how to handle life every day.
It's not fun and it's lonely.

April 5, 2017
The past few days have been so bad. Everything hurts. It's like I am walking on Legos, shin splints through my whole body, hot flashes, dizziness, headaches, chest heaviness, blurred vision, body chills, muscles weakness, and nausea. But I still have to continue with my life and take care of my sick little boy. I have to act like everything is ok and nothing hurts.

Walking around Target today, getting things to help my little guy feel better. I had to stop because the pain in my legs was so bad. I acted like I was looking at food on the shelves, because I can't show the pain I am in. If people want to say it's all in my head, I would gladly trade bodies with them for an hour.

When you see me, know that I am hiding so much more than you think. The pain, you can't see, the fight I struggle with because my body is at war with itself. No pity please. Just understanding instead of judgment. I would not wish this on my worst enemy. I will keep fighting and I will have good days. Today is not one of those days. Today I am fighting with everything I have just to take care of my youngest. As long as he sees me doing my best to take care of him and knows that mommy will do everything she can to get him something he needs, that's enough for me. I want my kids to see a mom, not a disease.

April 7, 2017

It's weeks like this I wish I did have a caregiver coming to help out. I can't seem to function. I hate that I can't take care of my youngest and he has to fend for himself on these days. It makes being a mom really hard.

April 8, 2017

It makes me so sad how much my health has gone downhill and how it has changed me. Makes me wonder if I hadn't pushed myself so hard those 8 months and listened to the Drs., would I be as bad as I am now?

Can't go back unfortunately. All I can do is learn to listen to my body and hope that one day I can get it under control. This life is not fun and I want to be able to enjoy it with my babies.

April 13, 2017

MRI results were not the best, but so glad I can put off surgery a bit longer. So hopefully rehab will help, and I can go a few more years without having to have another back surgery.

April 14, 2017

I've been having Dizziness and chest heaviness since Tuesday night.... Forgot I ran out of meds on Monday... Oops. Gotta go pick those up today. I can't be missing meds like this. I have to be on top of it because I have been sick way too much.

April 15, 2017

Everything hurts so bad. It's like I can feel every nerve and it's not pleasant. Almost like my skin is ripped off and it's all exposed.

April 25, 2017

First day wearing the back brace-half the day, little sore, so we will see how I do tomorrow. Praying it will help, along with rehab/chiro. I hate having to miss so much because my back keeps torturing me.

I don't understand why it's not getting any better. This is stupid to think, but sometimes I wish I was paralyzed just so I wouldn't have to feel the pain. I know… Awful.

April 27, 2017

Back pain, sore muscles from doing rehab, normal daily pain, woman pain... So ready to crawl into my bed.

April 28, 2017

Initial injury was June 1, 2010. It's been almost 7 years now and in the past couple months, it's gotten worse. At this point, I'd settle for 50% of this back pain to be gone. Hopefully, in the next 2 weeks, we will figure out the next steps.

May 3, 2017

I actually had some energy today and vacuumed, cleaned up the house a little, went for a short walk with my youngest.... I'm so exhausted now.

May 11, 2017

The amount of pain I'm in right now... Hurts so bad to walk and stand. All from walking the past couple days and rehab exercises. I'm over it and it needs to go away.

May 12, 2017

Getting packed up and ready to head out soon to get all the kids from school and then heading down to spend the weekend with the boys for Mother's Day!!! Baseball game, Prom, and mom/son time. I can't wait!!!

May 15, 2017

Took me a couple days to recover from Mother's Day weekend, but it was worth being able to be there for my oldest son's first Prom. He looked so handsome.
Going to EBJ on Thursday to see what they can do for my lower back. Hopefully the Dr. can fix the issue.

May 18, 2017

Funny how I'm right back here. Let's see what my Dr. can do this time. Surgery is in my near future. Hoping for the best outcome. We decided that since my back isn't getting any better, it might be best to do the fusion.

May 27, 2017

2am and sleep just isn't happening. Probably because parts of my body feel like they are on fire, while others are throbbing with pain and some parts have a prickly feeling through them. Headache and nausea just add that last little kick I need to keep me awake.

May 29, 2017

Omg I hate this pain. My body isn't gonna be able to take this much longer.

June 1, 2017

No motivation today. Tired, feeling worn down. Told myself to just get through a 30 min workout.... I did 55 min!!!!! Now I'm worthless for the rest of the day. I showered and put on sweats. Done for the day.

June 2, 2017

I feel like I was punched in the jaw. The whole right side of my face down into my neck hurts so bad.

June 3, 2017

I've gotta be up in 4 hours....... pain is keeping me awake. It's gonna be a rough day.

June 9, 2017

I definitely over did it today. But on the plus side, my house is clean!! Those who don't understand, this was a HUGE thing for my body to go through. Gonna be resting the rest of the night.

It's so sad that the little things that people do, like showering, can take me out for the rest of the day. It's really irritating, and I am jealous of all the healthy people.

June 11, 2017

It's days like today I really hate my body (mainly the low back), it's hurting so bad that I can't walk. The price I pay for hanging out with friends. I'm in bed, resting and praying the pain will go away enough for me to walk around.

I feel so bad for my youngest. I'm stuck in bed and can barely move. He has been entertaining himself, making his own lunch and snacks (even though he microwaved frozen raw hamburger patties), and checking on me to see if I need anything. This kid deserves an award.

June 14, 2017

Feeling the Addisons today. My youngest got his own dinner together and asked me if I wanted him to make me something to eat too. He is so sweet. I'm such a lucky mom. I'm not hungry at all and he is really trying to make me eat something. I know I should, but most days it's just too hard to eat anything.

June 21, 2017

Surgery was approved by insurance. Should hear back sometime soon about the surgery date.

Pre-op appointment is on Tuesday and then we will look at a time that works with my schedule for surgery. I really hope that it works this time. I am done with all this back pain. If I can get that fixed, maybe the Addison's and Fibro wouldn't be so bad.

June 26, 2017

So, my endocrinologist didn't like my blood sugar levels, so I have to go in early tomorrow and have blood drawn for a few different things. I am always bordering on being diabetic, so I need to do everything I can to keep me from becoming diabetic.

June 27, 2017

Got done with my pre-op appointment and so they will be sending all my blood work and EKG results to my Dr. tomorrow and once everything looks good, they will call, and I'll have a surgery date.

June 28, 2017

Today has been a struggle. Dizziness, fatigue, pain, and blurred vision. If my little guy will let me, I'm gonna head to bed and hopefully sleep and feel way better in the morning.

June 29, 2017

Just got the call. Surgery is August 1st, unless there is a cancellation.

I have a month to get my body in good shape for surgery. I want to have a healthy body to make it easier for healing time, so I really need to keep motivated. The pain and struggle it takes to get through some workouts will be worth it... I'm hoping. This will also help me compare pre and post-surgery workouts and what my body can handle after. This will help me know if the surgery was a success as well. Having the back pain gone will also help me know how to better handle my Addisons and Fibro flare ups. I'm very excited and scared at the same time. There is a chance I may not survive the surgery because of the stress it will cause to my body, but the pain I deal with on a daily basis, is not a life I enjoy living.

Got off the phone with my pre-op nurse. They did a nose swab and I have a staph infection but it's not contagious and I won't get sick or anything but have to take antibiotics and my iron levels were low, so I have to go in 3 times in 1 week for 2 hours and sit with an IV. And I was so happy because I thought all my results were good. Guess I don't know how to read bloodwork results correctly.

July 4, 2017

Talk about just the motivation I needed. Was running and doing a workout at the track. There were 2 soccer teams practicing and the coach of the high school team stopped me and asked if I was an athlete. Of course I laughed and said I used to be. He said him and his team were watching my workout and were really impressed with my athleticism. He asked if I ever coached or wanted too. I said I've never played soccer but thanks. He told me to keep it up because I'm doing a great job. Here I was thinking my workouts were wimpy and embarrassingly easy. That is just what I needed. Nothing beats getting complimented on your workouts from a stranger who is impressed with how you are trying to kill it.

July 5, 2017

Nothing like being in bed at 2pm because you're in so much pain from trying to enjoy the 4th. I feel bad that my youngest can't go out and enjoy today's sun because I can barely move.

I really think having a care giver would be fantastic.

July 6, 2017
When your ankles feel like they can't support your weight and your back pain is so bad you can barely lift your legs enough to walk, and your upper body feels like the bones are frozen and trying to defrost.... Yup, that's my current situation.
I don't understand why my body doesn't want to function. Well, I guess I do. It hates me and wants me dead.

July 8, 2017
2 hours at the festival.... I really need to invest in a wheelchair. That was a bit much for my body. I guess I don't realize how much pressure it puts on my low back, but I sure can feel it. My youngest had the best time and it always a joy to see him smiling and enjoying life.
I just wish all this pain would stop. If it's not the back, it's a flare. If it's not a flare, it's a cold. It's a never-ending cycle of pain and fatigue.
Surgery is soon and I am hopeful that it will all be great after.

July 11, 2017
It's so sad. I hope they find better treatments for Addisons. It's awful and painful and hard for people to understand.
I hate reading about people dying from Addisons. From not getting the right treatment when they go to the ER for a crisis. It really angers me, that there are so many ER doctors who don't know what Addison's is and they just dismiss it. Something needs to be done.

July 16, 2017
Today is one of those really bad days. I just feel bad for my youngest who has to suffer because I can't do anything. It's like my body is to heavy and my muscles are too weak to move it. Even though I want to move it, it just isn't cooperating.

July 17, 2017

Omg the pain I am feeling right now, it's like all my nerves are exposed. It hurts so bad and I just want it to stop. This is one of the worst kind of pains. This is the one that never stops, that makes you want to rip your own skin off. I sit and rock back and forth, praying it will end soon, but it doesn't.

Had to smoke and relax myself and hopefully I'll fall asleep before I rip my skin off.

July 19, 2017

Really Nurse??? You just looked at my chart and asked me what kind of infusion I'm getting and how much....

This fusion hurt so bad. I left, and I couldn't use my left arm all day. It was so achy and weak. I am not sure what they did, but it fucking hurts.

I have been tired and weak all day. I do not like what this iron fusion has done. It did not say that this would be one of the side effects.

July 20, 2017

Looking back at this point in my life, makes me sad. The one job I loved doing and was good at is now gone from my life. My body failed to keep up and I had to let it go. I miss it so much. I hate that this disease is taking so many things I love away from me. I try to stay positive, but some days are harder than others.

Just a couple more weeks and I will have the surgery and then everything will just start getting better.

July 23, 2017

Even though I am feeling like I was beaten and left for dead, yesterday was worth it. Time with the boys, making memories, family days.... worth the worst pain in the world.

I let my husband decide where to take me for a date night and he picks this...... gaming restaurant, as in nerd gaming (think dungeons and dragons). I can barely read the menu because it's all weird references. Interesting crowd, but he should have just brought one of his friends instead.

115

July 29, 2017

When you kick the door with all 4 small toes and the pain goes all the way to your hip.... Yep, that's how I started my morning.

The longer I have to be without meds that help me manage my pain, the harder it is. It has been so hard to sleep the last couple nights. I am in such horrible pain it hurts to just sit, lay, and be in bed. When I try to get up and walk, it hurts even more. 3 more days til my surgery and I can get back to trying to manage the pain. I am fatigued and just done with all of this. Can I be put to sleep until my surgery? I just want the pain to stop.

BACK SURGERY: ROUND 2

This summer I was watching our friend's kids. It was nice that my youngest had friends to play with and I didn't have to try to entertain him. My oldest was working and my middle son did a week on a week off. I was mentally trying to prepare myself for the surgery. I looked up YouTube videos on people who had L5S1 ALIF surgery to see how they were doing. I was not impressed, and it made me even more scared.

I sat down and wrote the boys letters. I wrote one out for their 18th bdays, graduations, wedding days, and for when they became parents-1 letter for each occasion to each boy, just in case I didn't make it through surgery.

I was really scared that I would die during surgery. I was scared my body wouldn't be able to handle the stress of it. I wasn't being over dramatic. When a common cold can kill you, surgery is a bit scarier.

Finally, August 1st was here. My dad came up, just in case this might be the last time he was able to see me. It was nice having him here. It was the first time him and my husband had met, and the first time I had seen him in 16 years. We talked on the phone, but never had the chance to see each other. He had just moved to Oregon, so he was only 5 hours away now.

I didn't sleep at all the night before surgery. I was so nervous and scared. I had to be at the hospital at 5am and surgery was scheduled for 7am.

I got to the room and the nurse was so funny. She had me laughing. I think she could tell I was nervous and wanted to help calm me. I had to wash up again, with that special soap and then get in the gown.

My husband and dad came back when they had the Drs. and anesthesiologist came to talk to me. The anesthesiologist was an ass. He kept telling me that I didn't need to stress dose for the surgery because there were no cases of people with Addisons disease who died in surgery from not stress dosing. Well duh!! Asshole, it's because they all stress dosed. For one, he didn't even know what Addisons disease was, so I am sure he was pulling that information out of his ass. He acted like he wasn't going to give me the hydrocortisone I needed for the surgery-even though my Endo STRESSED how important those dosages were, pre, during, and post-surgery.

They gave me something to relax me as they wheeled me away for surgery and I was asleep before we hit the elevators. I wish I could use whatever they gave me to relax at home for nights I can't sleep.

When I woke up, I felt so out of it. My throat was so dry, and my head was spinning. The nurse took a deep breath and said "Finally, you're awake." I was still trying to come out of it. She told me that they had been trying to wake me up for over an hour, and I wasn't responding. She was getting a little worried because I would stop breathing. Once she had me awake, she did some tests to see if I was ok.

This is where I got really scared. She told me to move my toes, so I started to wiggle my toes. Again, she said "move your toes." I told her I was. I looked down and could see that my toes were not moving at all. She ran a pen up my foot and there was no reaction, no flinch, nothing. I started to internally panic.

She stayed calm and told me she was going to get the Dr. He came and did the same thing she just did. He said the surgery went fine, so there is no reason my legs shouldn't be working. Really!! Then why are they not working??? He told her to stop the pain meds and see if that will help with getting movement back. Wait?? You just cut me open and now you want to stop the pain meds, so you can "see" if that is what is causing the lack of leg movement? I had to brace myself for the pain I knew would hit hard. Boy did it ever.

The pain was like labor that wouldn't stop. I could barely catch my breath and I was crying. Every time I moved it just made it worse. The good thing was, after about an hour, I was able to move my toes. That meant I could have the pain meds again. The bad news, the pain meds weren't cutting it once I got them. It took about 10 hours for them to kick in a take the pain away. I was so loopy, I don't remember some of the conversations I had had. Apparently, one was about Jennifer Lopez and I had my friends laughing so hard, which was painful for me when I started laughing.

I had in a catheter and I couldn't remember if I had actually gotten up to pee, or even felt like I had to pee. I told the nurse, "I haven't peed since I've been in recovery." She looked at my bag and said there was pee in it. "I haven't felt the urge to pee at all, why can't I feel myself going?" She thought that was weird as well, but we found out that it was normal. I guess it was the kind of catheter they did or something like that. I am not sure because I was so hopped up on meds.

I had to stay 2 nights, when I was supposed to go home that same day. I wasn't breathing when I would fall asleep, so they wanted to make sure I was stable enough to go home.

My Dr. came to see me on day 2 and asked why I still had the catheter in and why I hadn't gotten out of bed yet. I told him that I didn't know, I was just lying there waiting to hear when I could do all that. He said that he had put the orders in for the catheter to be removed when I got to the recovery room. He was almost yelling at the poor nurse who was in the room at the time. She had no clue what was going on, but she looked like she was going to cry, he was not happy. He showed me that the orders where put in, so someone just neglected to do it. He had them take it out and had the PT lady come in asap. He said that if she felt I was ok to go home after she watched me walk, then he would work on the discharge papers.

I was so happy. I just wanted to be home and in my own bed. She came in and showed me how to get up properly and I had to walk up 3 stairs. Which was nice because we have 3 stairs at the entry of our house. I was able to do it, with a lot of pain, but it was done and now I could go home.

I was thankful that my friend took time off work to come help me out for a couple days. My husband couldn't take the time off, so it was nice that my friends rallied together to help. People came and dropped food off, so I didn't have to cook. Some friends sent food to the house.

The boys were here to help out and I was still watching all the kids, so they were also helping as much as they could.

I had to sit and do nothing for 4 weeks. So, I binged watched *Grey's Anatomy*. I was spiraling into a deeper depression that I was trying to ignore. I had so much bloating and I wasn't using the bathroom. The stool softeners weren't working, so I added in some smooth move tea. That did it. I was peeing shit so bad, all day. My asshole was on fire. I was in so much pain that it hurt to sit. Then shit just started falling out. I couldn't believe I shit my pants at 37 years old. I was just glad no one was around to see it…. that time.

The next day, when my friend was visiting me, she was about to leave, and I was sitting in the chair, and shit poured out of my ass. I was so glad she was leaving, because I was mortified. I don't know what I would have done if she was staying. I hope she didn't smell it. If she did, she was polite and didn't say a thing. I wanted to die.

I had so much time to sit and think about things, it was not good. I broke down one day and cried for an hour. My dog came and comforted me, she didn't leave my side.

My sister came over and I broke down again. She reassured me that this was temporary. That I would be good, I just had to give myself time to heal. It had only been 3 weeks, and healing time might take up to a year.

I went in for a few post-op checkups. I was thrilled when I got the go ahead to walk a bit outside. I had to use a walker and my youngest would go on little 5 min walks with me. I didn't make it far in those 5 minutes, but I did that a couple times a day.

In September I decided to do the Vegetarian/seafood diet thing and stick with it. I had put on 35 lbs. and I was not happy. I knew that it had been from the meds and from being inactive, but I was looking at the surgery as a new start. I watched all the documentaries about food on Netflix and thought, shit... I'll go vegan, but with fish. So, I started my veganish-seafood diet.

I went in again in October and got the go ahead to walk some more, but not to push myself. It was so hard. I wanted to go all out and see what my body could handle. I was feeling better. There was not a lot of pain. I was walking more and slowly getting out of my depression (or so I tried to tell myself). I was thankful that I was seeing a therapist and was able to talk through some of it, but I think I was still lying to myself.

Journal Entry: August 2017- February 2018

August 4, 2017

Talk about having to suck up your pride. My poor husband had to shower me and put lotion on me. I feel like everything I say or ask for is a demand. I really can't do anything by myself. So grateful for those who have stepped up to help because this sucks.

August 5, 2017

Hit myself in the stomach twice last night. Ended up tucking my hands under me so I wouldn't do it again. Then had a dream I was playing basketball and jumped in the dream, which made me jolt, so that was painful. It's been a high pain kind of day so far.

August 6, 2017

Boys took me for a walk outside today. I was able to walk about 200 meters with the walker, so that's good. Taking myself off pain meds, but that is what is making things hard. Trying to only take the oxy at night so I can sleep and Tylenol once a day with the muscle relaxer. Hopefully by mid-week I won't need any of it.

Boys had me laughing, which hurt. They were being so weird, but it was worth the pain. Dancing around to Mexican music, saying "It's all in the hips." My middle son was dancing around and said, "look at my chest brah," and would start pumping his chest up and down. They were being comedians and little weirdos and it made my night, I love them so much. They are crazy and wild, just like their mom. Can't wait til we can all dance around crazy with each other.

August 7, 2017

My body is telling me I over did it yesterday and it's not happy at all. Who would have thought tiny walks could cause so much pain? I know it's only been a week, but I want my body to heal faster.

August 10, 2017

It's getting harder to sit here and do nothing. I'm going stir crazy. I want to go out and walk and get my body moving. Yes, I get that I need rest and time to heal but it is driving me crazy. I've never been home this long without going anywhere. I'm going insane!!!

August 12, 2017

I'm amazed at how animals just know things. Haelee knows and she watches me and looks out for me. She is the best dog, maybe a bit too protective of her kids against Skky (my other dog), but I'm so glad she is my little girl.

August 17, 2017

Went for a walk today. About 1/2 mile. Definitely feeling it, but if I can do that every day for a few days, I'm sure I won't be as sore and tired.

August 20, 2017

That was a bit much, so I know my body can only go about 20 min. So maybe 2-20 min walks a day should be good. This recovery is taking forever. Addisons and fibro really slow down the healing process.

August 23, 2017

Did about 20 min on the elliptical, because my feet started to go numb, so I knew it was time to stop. But it felt good otherwise.
Did 10 wall ball squats and some light leg stretching. It's small but it's a good start.

August 25, 2017

Past 3 days I've wanted to tear off my own skin. The pain has been so bad, it's like my entire body has a horrible burn and I can't get rid of the pain.

The only relief I got was when I took a hot shower. It's made sleeping almost impossible. I just want it to go away.

Decided to smoke so the pain would subside. I hate my body so much.

September 7, 2017

Been awake since 3am. Not feeling good and not sleeping is a bad combo. Hoping this cold doesn't get worse.

Eating some bananas, drinking coconut water, gonna have butternut squash soup for dinner tonight. Hopefully I'll feel better tomorrow. I don't have time to be sick. I feel like today was wasted, but I'm resting so my body can heal faster.

September 11, 2017

I think I found a big trigger to my pain. Felt good (despite the cold sickness) for 3 days. I was eating only veggies, fruit, quinoa and seafood. Yesterday I decided to try spelt bread with avocado, a smoothie with gluten free granola and then later for dinner had veggie burger on a gluten free bun. Later that night I had excruciating leg and hip pain and pain in my upper joints as well. I believe wheat is a no go. Staying away from that and seeing how I feel and then I will try to add wheat back in and see what happens.

September 16, 2017

Went shopping, got some juicing done, made shrimp salad for the party tonight, made some chocolate avocado pudding and homemade coconut whipped cream.

My body is hurting right now. Resting til the pain subsides a bit. Being on my feet for 3 hours is more than I can handle. It really hurt my back being up that much, as well as the rest of my body. It's been over a month, so I should not be feeling like this still.

September 18, 2017

I go in on Thursday for my 2nd post-op appointment. In my head he will tell me I can go running and exercise again, and I'll be able to return to bending, twisting, lifting and driving long distances. I'm not ready for reality, but I'm sure I'll be unhappy with what he says unless it's what I want him to say.

September 20, 2017

Today is amazing because I am released to normal activity!!!! Well as long as it doesn't cause pain and I slowly go into it, but it's a go. He said it all looks solid and if I can do exercises and running without pain, then it's a success. I will slowly ease back in, but I am just so happy right now. The hard part is going to be taking it easy and not trying to push myself to my limits.

September 21, 2017

I have been struggling with fatigue today. So hard to keep my eyes open and move around. Can it be bedtime yet?
Suffering: A good word for what I am going through. Along with the things that come with pain or have caused me to get the autoimmune disease (and all the ones that will continue to pile on). I have to stay positive. I can't keep falling into this depression.

September 25, 2017

Today has been a bad fatigue day. I've done nothing and struggled to keep my eyes open all day.
My stomach is still hurting from the bulge that showed up on Saturday, on the scar where the surgery was. I'm having it looked at on Wednesday. Seems it's just 1 thing after the other.

September 26, 2017

So happy I am getting this lump looked at tomorrow. It is starting to hurt even worse. Every step I take it causes pain in that area. I am so scared that they are going to have to go in again and fix this. I don't want to have to be cut open again.

September 27, 2017

Went into the Dr. and he is confused at what the lump is. It's not acting like a hernia, but it is at the same time. He says it's in an odd place to be a hernia and it's hard and it won't push back in. But when I lay down it disappears and comes back out when I stand up. He is gonna talk to another Dr. who deals with this stuff and then let me know what steps to take. The good news is, is that I can go for runs and workout as long as it's not strenuous on my lower abdominals.

I just need to be happy that I am released to run. Now I can run off this depression.

October 1, 2017

On September 1st, I started my big diet change due to having too many flares. It has been an amazing change for me. I am doing a plant-based diet with seafood (think vegan). I am not having any bread with gluten. I tried having some and I had a flare up (could have been the spelt bread or the wheat in the veggie burger-Not 100% sure, but I will try gluten free noodles this week), so I decided to just take it out.

I am really surprised that I have not been missing all the other foods. I love that in 1 month I have only had 2 days of a flare up, when it was 4-6 a week (granted I am still fatigued and have fibro/Addison pain from being cold or over doing it-but the food flare pain was the worst for me.) I am really glad I decided to do this. Now I just have to manage the other pains and I should be good.

Unfortunately, the amazing Pad Thai I had tonight has caused a flare up. I am not sure what it was in it that caused the flare (I am thinking it was the brown sugar since I haven't had that type of sugar since August), but I will not be making it again.

October 2, 2017

Great. Every step I take with my right foot is now making my lump hurt. Good thing I go in first thing tomorrow. It also is poking out more and feels bigger.

I hate that my body just can't do one thing that is normal. Just let yourself heal perfectly. That is all I am asking. I don't want to have to keep going through weird shit every few months.

October 3, 2017

Gonna wait for the phone call from my Dr. to confirm about the lump before I believe what the tech told me. I'm glad it's not serious, painful, but nothing I can't handle.

The Dr. called and said it is nothing to worry about. It will go away, but if it gets worse, I need to come in. I guess I will just pray that it goes away quickly, because the pain it is causing with walking is really annoying and it is hindering my workouts.

October 12. 2017

This cold weather is not good for my body. Past couple days have been hell. I need some sun and warmth. It feels like my body is frozen and trying to defrost. You know that pain when you grab something really cold and then it takes your hand a while to warm up, but that pain the cold causes it? Ya, that's how my whole body feels.

October 14, 2017

Haven't been able to do anything like this with the boys in about 7 years. My youngest was so excited for me to join them at the trampoline park. I only did 30 min of the 90 min session they had, but it was so much fun to finally be able to join and not just watch.

Not sure how my body will handle that much play, but I hope that it does good and won't cause me to be in too much pain later.

October 16, 2017

My body is still trying to recover from all the activities from Saturday at the trampoline park. I had plans for today, but my diseases had another. So, it looks like I'm resting all day instead.

October 21, 2017

Drove down for my oldest son's homecoming night. I was already in so much pain when I left, it was hard to keep it together. The mix of the drive, being so cold, and sitting in the hard bleachers was way too much on my body. It was worth seeing him and his girlfriend win Homecoming king and queen.

October 22, 2017

Every part of me hurts. I was able to get 3½ hours of sleep, but the pain kept waking me. Walking is not an option today, so I will be in my bed resting, if I can. It may take me a few days to recover, but the pain and fatigue is worth being there for special moments. I'm so grateful that my youngest understands when mommy has bad days and just needs to rest. He's great at taking care of me.

Missed half of the bday party, but so glad I was able to get myself up. Got home and put on jammies and crashed again. My body is just not liking me doing anything.

October 23, 2017

Got my blood results back and I'm low in protein, potassium, and vitamin D. Some diet adjustments and hopefully I'll be able to figure it all out.

Not a lot of people understand my illness, and I don't expect them too. Nor do I care that people think I'm "faking" or "wanting attention", because if they really knew me and who I am, those thoughts wouldn't even cross their mind. I don't want sympathy either. I was dealt this card, so I am dealing with it the best I can.

I will do what I can, when I can. I don't need to explain myself. My family and friends understand and are supportive and that's all I need. If people want to be judgy and be hateful, by all means, I will let them hold onto that hate, because it doesn't impact me. Just makes me sad for them.

October 26, 2017

Left for Vegas. Brought my wheelchair with me just in case. We will see how my body will be able to handle this trip.

Already stressing so much about the plane ride, but I did stress dose today, so I think it should be good.

October 30, 2017

I'm so excited to see my baby boy. Just wish I felt better. Had so much fun in Vegas and I can't wait to do it again next year. Even though it was really rough on me and I left every party early, I still enjoyed myself. I was glad my husband and friends stayed out and partied. I hated to be the Debbie Downer and leave everything, but my body just couldn't handle it all.

One night I got really sick from the food we ate. I barely made it back to the hotel room, before I was spewing out of both ends.

November 1, 2017

Felt bloated and had gas. On the verge of fast potties. Had some energy but felt fatigued. Got hungry but didn't stop to eat.

Went to EBJ for my 3-month post-op. No restrictions, and the lump is feeling better. I am so glad I will be able to do whatever I want in my workouts. Still have to take it easy and not push too hard though.

Therapy went great and decided to start this food journal to help me eat and track my body/food stresses.

Started rearranging the house. Didn't need to workout because moving furniture was a great workout. Had some joint pain (from moving stuff) and nausea.

9:40am-Banana

11:45am-Strawberry/banana smoothie with rice milk, pecans and almond butter

12:15pm- 4 mini KitKats

6pm- Rice, broccoli and edamame
8:30pm- 2 mini tootsie rolls and 2 small bags of skittles
3½ bottles of water

November 2, 2017

Felt good. Energized and by 8pm I was tired enough to fall asleep. Had
some LB pain, but that was from moving furniture and stuff around.
Started spotting with some light cramps. Got the house done.
Boys were texting me, letting me know they were on their way to State CC.
Used moving the rooms around as my workout again.
Joint pain again from moving stuff.

8:20am- banana
12:30pm- hash browns
3pm- sweet potato chips
3:30pm- 3 mini snickers, 3 tootsie rolls
5:30pm- edamame
5 bottles of water

November 3, 2017

Felt good today. Slept well, but needed an afternoon nap, after I ate lunch.
Felt tired all day. Drove to Pasco and had to eat in the car. Pain all over
from driving.
Felt really sick at the hotel. Spotting and cramps.

9am- banana
12:30pm- grits
2:30pm- 3 mini KitKats
5:35pm- sweet potato chips, carrots with hummus
5 bottles of water

November 4, 2017

Stomach has been iffy all day from eating off the diet. Gassy and slight pain. Body aches/pain from the drive. I feel dehydrated, tired, sluggish. Combo of food and traveling.

Cramps got worse, so I had to take ibuprofen. Spotting was the same but should have worn a pad.

8:45am- white hot chocolate, gluten free ham and egg english muffin (*Starbucks*)
1pm- gas station burrito
5:45pm- edamame
3 bottles of water

November 5, 2017

Felt a bit sluggish today and tired. Woke up at 6:30am and couldn't fall back asleep. Little nauseous all day and some cramping. LB pain was at a level 3 as well as body pain.

8:30am- strawberry/banana smoothies with rice milk, pecans, and almond butter
11:45am- avocado toast with sriracha
1:45pm- 1 mini KitKat, 2 mini snickers
3:45pm- sushi
4:45pm- ¼ large popcorn (movie theater)
4 bottles of water

November 6, 2017

Felt good most of the day. A little tired, but not enough to slow me down. Hit a wall about 5:30pm. No body pain (besides cramps). Feeling bloated from period (stared November 2nd-mostly spotting). Worked out with no pain.

Would be nice if the spotting would stop. Not sure if it is something I should be worried about. I guess if it lasts more then 10 days, I'll have it checked out.

8:10am- toast with butter
10:15am- grits
1:40pm- edamame
3:40pm- 4 mini M&M bags
6pm- 5 tacos
7 bottles of water

November 7, 2017

Felt good again today. Did yoga and had no pain. Around 5pm started getting really gassy. Felt tired all day, but not exhaustion.

8:15am- toast with PB
10:30am- potatoes with onions
12:50pm- smoothies (nut)
3:50pm- baby carrots
5:50pm- tilapia, rice, and edamame
6 bottles of water

November 8, 2017

Extremely exhausted today. I could have slept all day. No pain, just super fatigued and wiped out. Had doxepin the night before, so it could be that.

8:30am- PB toast
9:30am- grits
12:40pm- edamame
5:30pm- 5 tacos
5 bottles of water

November 9, 2017

Hurting really bad after the long drive all the way down to get the boys. Pain was at a 9. Legs felt restless and painful. Joints felt like they were going to swell so big they would explode. My oldest was worried about me being in that much pain and was trying to get us home quickly.

9:30am-PB toast
11:30am- sweet potato chips
3:30pm- sweet potato chips
7:30pm- banana
8:30pm- popcorn

November 10, 2017

Felt like I had some energy. Had a spark around 11am. Took all my vitamins. Some LB pain but it was a 2 and about a 4-leg pain towards the end of the night. Only got 4 hours of sleep the night before. Ran around a lot, but it was a pretty good day pain wise. Was able to bake cookies without being too exhausted.

7:50am- PB toast
3:20pm- chips
5:30pm- rice, shrimp, and asparagus
8:30pm- chocolate chip vegan cookie
4 bottles of water

November 11, 2017

Felt some back pain. Right hand had a hard time gripping and squeezing. It was hard to put on Chapstick and squeeze the contact solution. Did not do good eating today.
Level 4 body pain and level 6 leg pain. Legs and hips were hurting after sitting through the movie.
Tired but not exhausted. Started adrenal support and bio plasm salt today.

8:45am- banana
9:30am- hash browns
1:30pm- oriental salad
4:15pm- 2 protien balls, pistachios
6:15pm- spaghetti
7pm- ¼ large movie theater popcorn
5 bottles of water

November 12, 2017

Felt good, but tired. Level 3 overall pain.

8:20am- banana
12:30pm- oriental salad
6pm- tofu spinach, Brussel sprouts over rice.

November 13, 2017

Felt good. Got in a workout. Little stressed dealing with my youngest's teeth (his middle brother chipped off his bottom 2 front teeth playing with his Beyblades), but got it all done. Level 2 pain all over. Not overly tired, but hit a wall around 6pm, which is good.

8:40am- banana
1:30pm- oriental salad
5:30pm- red potatoes, asparagus, Brussel sprouts and tilapia
5 bottles of water

November 14, 2017

Felt good again. LB pain while doing yoga.
After sitting for a while, I got up to move around and my legs felt like they were swelling to the verge of popping. Didn't feel tired until about 7:30pm.

8:45am- PB toast
11am- 2 protein balls
12:45pm- 5 tacos
6pm- leftovers
5 bottles of water

November 15, 2017

Only slept for 4 hours. Was up at 5am. Tired but made it through the day without feeling like I needed a nap. Sore from yoga, but no body pain. Overall it was a good health day.

7:45am- PB toast
12pm- 2 protien bites mean green
2:15pm- 3 pieces of avocado toast- 2 protein bites
5:35pm- mean green
5:50pm- 2 pieces of PB toast- 1 slice pizza
6 bottles of water

November 16, 2017

Very tired this morning. Got up and ate then went back to bed and slept for an hour. Still felt tired and wanted to nap around 1pm but didn't. Just feel worn down.
LB had sharp pain in an isolated area. No fibro pain. Slept almost 7 hours last night.

8:40am- PB toast
12:30pm- chips and avocado
3pm- 2 protien bites
5:30pm- spinach, artichoke, quinoa casserole
8:10pm- 1 protien bite
5 bottles of water

November 17, 2017

Felt good today. No pain with workout. Had energy. Didn't feel like I needed a nap. I don't think I had any pain. Could have drank more water. Took doxepin and melatonin to help with sleep tonight. Down to 149lbs. Slept almost 7 hours.

8:30am- PB toast
11am- 2 protein bites
12:30pm- 5 tacos
6:15pm- broccoli, rice, tofu
3 bottles of water

November 18, 2017

Slept til 10:30am. Tired all day but pushed myself to do a workout. Was only going to do 15 min but did 1 hour.

Got some energy around 2pm. Went to *Costco* and *Half Price Books*. Got my youngest a book. Walked around *Target*. Around 5:30pm I got really tired. At 6:30pm was having hard time keeping my eyes open when I was sitting on the couch.

Tried to do a movie night with my little guy, but he was not into it. Trying to keep myself awake, so I walked around.

Pain was very low today. Some mild LB pain, sore from workout. Very exhausted but I think it was mostly from the doxepin. That is one thing I really hate about the doxepin, it helps you sleep, but makes you a zombie the next day. I already struggle with fatigue, I don't need that added on too.

12:30pm- 2 pieces of PB toast
2pm- mean green
3:50pm- 4 protien bites
5:15pm- 5 tacos
6:45pm- popcorn
5 bottles of water

November 19, 2017

Slept til 10am. I was really tired when I got up at 7:30am but was able to fall back asleep. My body must have needed the extra rest. Besides exhaustion and feeling like I was moving in slow motion, I didn't feel like I had Addison/fibro pain. Some low back pain with bending.

Stressed over my husband's behavior and having to answer the questions my youngest had about it. It's getting ridiculous and I hate that my youngest has to see his dad so angry so quickly over little things.

I am feeling extra stressed and I'm wondering if that has anything to do with how exhausted I am. I don't want to spend all day in bed, but maybe that is exactly what my body is needing. I feel I'm falling off good eating habits. Too much snacking and not enough eating good meals.

10:40am- 5 protein bites
12:30pm- mean green and banana

1pm- popcorn
2:15pm- sweet potato chips- 2 protien bites
5:45pm church Thanksgiving dinner. Rolls, veggies, mashed potatoes.
8:30pm- 1 bag (8) protien balls
4 bottles of water

November 20, 2017

Was woken up at midnight from my husband playing the Xbox, (loudly) and couldn't fall back asleep til almost 3am. Little man woke me up at 5am and I couldn't fall back asleep until after 7:30am. Slept til 10am. Felt run down and exhausted but had to push through.

Went and got a ring put in my nose, *Costco* for meds, *Trader Joes*, and *Target* for groceries. Skky took off at some point in the am and I had to go get her from the shelter.

My body is sore from working out the other day. I took today off from working out. I felt like I could have slept all day. I didn't have fibro pain, just the exhaustion. Took some melatonin to help ease me into sleep. I need to get back on track for my schedule. The fatigue has had me beaten since Friday.

10:40am- banana
1:15pm- grits
1:45pm- mean green
3:30pm- 1 bag (8) protien bites
5:30pm- 2 pieces of avocado toast
8pm- chips
3 bottles of water

November 21, 2017

Got up at 7:15am. Another outburst of anger from my husband, so my youngest asked me to take him to school because he was too scared to go with his dad. I made him anyways and reassured him it was ok. My husband blows up at the little stuff, but I know that he would never hurt me or my boys, he just has a childlike tantrum way too much. Not the best way to start the day.

Did a workout and upped the weights. Felt good to work off the stress from this morning's little tantrum. Went to therapy and got to talk through how bad the last week has been. Low back pain was at a level 3 today. Mostly from the workout.

Felt like I had good energy today. No fibro or Addison's pain.

Applied for a job with *3010 Weight Loss* to see if I can make it on my own. I don't want to stress like this anymore, but I need to do what's right for the boys, whether it's staying or leaving, but I also can't continue with the stress of this marriage either. I thought we would be able to make this work, but he stresses me out way more than anything else.

8:25am- banana
10:30am- 2 protien bites
1pm- fried tofu with soy sauce
3:45pm- pistachios
6pm- 4 slices of pizza
4 bottles of water

November 22, 2017

Had pain in joints last night when I was in bed. I think it was from the cheese on the pizza. Didn't fall asleep until after 2am. Only slept for 4 hours.

During the day I was ok. Still some joint pain but forced myself to clean the house and I did a 20 min elliptical/resistance session. Felt like I had energy all day. Pain was at a level 5, but I wasn't exhausted. Most of my pain was in the elbows and knees, really achy.

I need to work so I can feel useful and have my own thing, but I also know that I have way too many bad days, and no employer is going to hold onto someone who isn't reliable.

9:30am- PB toast
12:15pm- protien bites and banana
4:20pm- pistachios
5:50pm- shrimp
2 bottles of water

November 23, 2017

Got about 3½ hours of sleep last night. I can feel my body being affected by it. I need to get sleep. Up cooking all day. The pain in my legs and feet are pretty bad. Low back pain was at a level 6. I had the energy to make it through the day though. All over pain is about a 6 as well. Took doxepin and melatonin to help. Only took 2 doxepin, so hopefully I won't be to exhausted tomorrow.

10am- 2 pieces of PB toast
1:45pm- mean green- 1 protien bite- chips
5:30pm- Thanksgiving dinner
6:30pm- vegan pumpkin pie and vegan whipped cream
2 bottles of water

November 24, 2017

Got 9 hours of sleep and it was good sleep. Woke up but felt exhausted (from the doxepin), but got out of bed and did a workout. Woke me up more. Body pain was at a 3 today. I was tired, but I tried not to let it affect me. Hit a wall at 7pm and felt like I needed to go to bed. Had a glass of wine to see if it would cause a flare. I hope not, but I'll know later tonight or tomorrow.

9:20am- PB toast
1:30pm- turkey sandwich
5:30pm- sweet potato casserole
8:30pm- turkey sandwich and chips
5 bottles of water

November 25, 2017

Got 4 hours of sleep but felt rested. Laid in bed til 9am. Did a good hour workout and stretching. Went to *Target* and had to use the wheelchair. My body did not have a good day. Having a lot of nerve type pain in the legs, around the joints, and LB pain is a level 6. I didn't feel exhausted. I had enough energy and didn't even feel tired. I definitely know that I can't have wine now. I think that's why my body isn't doing well today. Hopefully I can get to bed before 2am. Also, not eating right is playing a big part in how shitty I have been feeling too. Around 10pm my body started to hurt really bad. Smoked to help with the pain. Trigger: sweet potato casserole- it has brown sugar in it...Brown sugar is a HUGE trigger for my flares.

9:20am- PB toast
12:30pm- turkey sandwich
3:30pm- protien bites
5:30pm- popcorn
5:45pm- bowl of sweet potato casserole
4 bottles of water

November 26, 2017
Felt like I slept good last night, got 6 hours in. Still a little rough waking up and getting moving. The pain was so bad last night. I think it affected my body today. Like it was still trying to recover.
Body was about a level 3 pain today. Felt pain through my joints every time I went outside. I really wish my body would just heal and I can go back to my life before 2010. 7 years of hell is long enough.

9:50am- PB toast
12:30pm- olives and chips
3pm- turkey, stuffing, potatoes, 2 rolls
5:30pm- pumpkin pie with whipped cream (vegan)
4 bottles of water

November 27, 2017
Today was a good day. I only got 4 hours of sleep, but I woke up with energy.
Did a workout, got everything on my list done.
There is soreness from working out and only had low back pain when I was bending. Made the decisions to pull my youngest from school and homeschool him. The stress of him struggling, having accidents all the time, and not getting his work done is way beyond what my body can handle right now.

Having some slight joint pain that is going up the arms, not sure why, but it's only a level 2 pain. Hoping to sleep good tonight.

8:30am- PB toast
10:30am- 2 pieces of PB toast
12:45pm- grits
3pm- popcorn
6pm- salmon, rice, Brussel sprouts
5 bottles of water

November 28, 2017

Woke up at 7:45am to my youngest in my bed and my husband still asleep. He had to leave for school at 8am. I rushed him and had him all ready for school in 8 mins.

Despite the rushing around this morning, my body did good today. Good energy and not painful (a level 2 pain). I do need to start getting more than 4 hours of sleep though. My body needs the rest. I really worry that lack of sleep is going to cause more harm to my body.

8:30am- PB toast
12:30pm- sushi and edamame
6pm- 5 tacos
3 bottles of water

November 29, 2017

Got 5 hours of sleep last night. 3rd night in a row that my little guy has come to my bed at around 5-6am.

Today was my rest day, which means I did some light house work. At around 5pm my body stared to hurt; feet, legs, and hips. I think it was from the hot chocolate and walking around. Seems the combo was not good for me. No more *Starbucks* for me.

8:45am- PB toast
9am- venti white hot chocolate- soy and peppermint
12pm- 2 protien bites

1:30pm- leftover salmon, rice and Brussel sprouts
2:15pm- chips and avocado
6:15pm- shrimp with almond, spaghetti noodles, zucchini with almonds
4 bottles of water

November 30, 2017

Got 5 hours of sleep last night. Woke up with some energy. Worked out and stayed on schedule. Low back pain has been at a level 3. No body pain early in the day. I stood up after sitting for a while and my left foot felt like my middle toe broke a blood vessel. Hurts to put any pressure on it. So strange. Hoping it goes away soon.

8:30am- PB toast
12:30pm- left over from dinner
5:30pm- 4 slices of pizza
4 bottles of water

December 1, 2017

My youngest sons 1st day of homeschool went ok. Got a lot to prepare and figure out so I can still get what I need to get done.

Got in a very short workout, which is ok, since I had to drive to my middle son's game. Took 3 hours to get there. By the 90 min mark, my body had had enough. Then having to sit on the hard bleachers. So glad it only took 70 min to get home.

My body is at a level 7 pain. I'm exhausted, but I know my mind won't let me sleep. I have too much to prepare for this coming week that it will keep me awake.

8:30am- PB toast
12pm- avocado Toast
2pm- handful of pistachios
5:20pm- seafood salad and imitation crap from *Safeway*
2 bottles of water

December 2, 2017

Was so exhausted from yesterday. Slept til 9am, got up and took my meds and ate, then went back to bed til 11:30am.

Had my youngest play the *Xbox* so I could rest. Got up and got some of his school stuff organized and a schedule set up. I was so exhausted, so I wasn't able to do much though. Wasn't hungry either.

I need good rest tonight, so I can get things done tomorrow.

Had some low back pain, but I think it's from sitting all day. Gotta move my body tomorrow so I don't get in a habit of not moving again.

9:30am- cereal
12:45pm- seafood salad
3pm- chips
6:25pm- handful of pistachios
4 bottles of water

December 3, 2017

Had more energy today. Body pain was at a level 5. Walking around the mall, my right leg was having some weird pain. Standing around in stores was killing my back and legs. Sucks that being out, walking around, is so painful. Was on my feet cleaning all day too.

9:15am- PB toast
12:15pm- protein bites
6pm- stir fry with tofu
3 bottles of water

December 4, 2017

Had a hard time getting up this morning. Didn't fall asleep til after 1 am. Got out of bed at around 8am and worked out but struggled through it. Struggling to find a balance between my day and homeschooling, but I'll get it down.

My low back was hurting today (about a level 3 pain and after my youngest son had his 2 hour practice, the pain is at a 7). I need to find a comfortable sleeping position to help alleviate the pain. I need a good solid-motionless 8 hours of sleep. Hopefully tomorrow will be better.

I also need to start eating better. It's hard when you don't really have an appetite, but I need to force myself to eat.

12:30pm- 3 tacos
4pm- vegan chocolate chip cookies
5:30pm- edamame
9pm- chips
4 bottles of water

December 5, 2017

Had a hard time getting up. Took ibuprofen last night to help with pain-but still slept really bad. Low back was about a level 4 today. Had some fibro pain but only about a level 2. Felt like I could have slept all day and probably should have rested, but things needed to be done. Went to therapy and talked about how I need to slow myself down in order to stop having so many flares.

Super exhausted and in pain- not taking anything, but gonna use the CBD.

9am- PB toast
12:30pm- ½ bowl of grits
2:30pm- avocado and chips
6:15pm- butternut squash
3 bottles of water

December 6, 2017

So cold last night, I couldn't get warm. Had to turn on the bed heater but didn't warm up for what seemed like forever. Slept crappy.

Hard time getting going. Felt tired all day. Laundry and vacuuming got done in spite of how lazy I wanted to be.

Fatigue and pain started about 6pm. The pain keeps getting worse. Not sure if I was stressed today, overdid it, ate something, or a combo; but the pain is at a level 8.

I took doxepin (1) to see if it helps and won't leave me feeling drugged tomorrow. I'm not sure I'll be able to sleep with this much pain though.

8:40am- PB toast
12pm- guac with tortillas
5:30pm- shrimp, green beans, and rice
7:30pm- vegan ice cream and chocolate chip cookie
5 bottles of water

December 7, 2017

Woke up feeling rested, but so cold. Fire died sometime in the early am and it was so cold throughout the house. I got 7 hours of motionless sleep though.
Didn't feel drugged when I woke up- so taking 1 doxepin should do the trick. My body was at about a level 2 pain and my back was at a 4.

8:30am- PB toast
12:15pm- 4 tacos
6pm- tilapia, Brussel sprouts, carrots, and rice
4 bottles of water

December 8, 2017

Got 5 hours of sleep last night. Struggled with energy today. LB pain was sharp when I would bend (about a 3-pain level). When I went outside I noticed joint pain that lingered for about an hour.
So exhausted tonight which I know means I won't sleep well. Stressing about my youngest son's birthday party and having all the people in the house. Here's hoping I can sleep tonight.

8:30am- PB toast
12pm- leftovers from last night's dinner
6:30pm- edamame
8pm- popcorn and 1 peppermint pattie
4 bottles of water

December 9, 2017
Gonna have to do this day on only 4 hours of sleep.
Got everything ready, cleaned, and set up for my little guys party. Was tired before it started.
Body did ok til about 3pm. Walking around *Bobakhan* and standing there was painful on my legs, hips, and low back. My feet started to hurt towards the end of the night. If I'm up standing, that's when I start to really hurt.

9am- PB toast
12:30pm- vegan pizza
1pm- bunt cake
4pm- pizza (little Caesars)
4 bottles of water

December 10, 2017
Felt exhausted but wanted to take advantage of the sun. I went for a 17 min run. Stretched and then sat for a while. Couldn't get motivated to get up after that.
Finally got up and showered. Struggling to do anything today and I am so ready for bed. Body pain has been a level 4 all day.

9am- PB toast
1pm- chips
3pm- edamame, angel roll, da bomb roll
5pm- avocado and chips
8:30pm- peppermint patties
4 bottles of water

December 11, 2017
Really tired all day. Brain fog at its best (felt stupid all day). My back has been hurting at a level 5.
Worked out and tried stretching my back, but it didn't help. Had to sit on the cement stairs for 2 hours at my youngest son's basketball practice, which made my back pain jump to an 8.

I feel like I could have slept all day. I don't know how I'm gonna get sleep, but I really need it tonight.

8:30am- PB toast
11am- banana
12:15pm- 5 tacos
5:30pm- salmon, asparagus, rice with almonds
2 bottles of water

December 12, 2017
Had to get up at 7:15am to get my youngest to his dentist appointment at 8am.
Went to therapy, picked up prescriptions, and to the bank to deposit a check. My youngest had his appointment with Dr. K to get his referral for ABA and speech therapy. When we got home we had to turn around and leave for Olympia. Watched my oldest son's basketball game and had to use my cushioned seat (it helped). Used one for driving too and that helped a lot. Was so exhausted all day. My back was at a level 8 pain. I hardly ate and was going on only 4 hours of sleep. I honestly don't know how I did anything today.

9:30am- PB toast
7pm- small bag of popcorn and snickers.
2 bottles of water

December 13, 2017
Exhausted all day. Pretty sore this morning and all day about a level 7 pain. I need to sleep good. I'm starting to feel like a zombie. Took 1 doxepin at 10pm. Maybe I can get enough sleep to be good for Friday's long drive, game, and drive back home. My body needs to do some major healing and with me only getting 3-5 hours of sleep each night, it's not happening.

9:30am- PB toast
2:30pm- tofu
5:30pm- asparagus with shrimp and couscous
5 bottles of water

December 14, 2017

Super exhausted all day. Fighting to just keep my eyes open. Low back pain was better (about a level 5). Can't wait to get in bed and hopefully get some sleep. Even a few hours would be nice.

8:45am- PB toast
12pm- leftover dinner
5:30pm- potato/Brussel sprout medley
7:15pm- almond joy cookies
5 bottles of water

December 15, 2017

Slept for 3 hours. Was awake for 30 min, slept another 3 hours. Got my youngest son done with school and drove down to watch the boys basketball game. Sitting in the bleachers was more bearable with the cushion.

8:30am- 2 PB toast
12pm- leftover dinner
3:30pm- pretzels
9pm- pretzels
11:45pm- 2 almond joy cookies
2 bottles of water

December 16, 2017

Body was ok today as far as Fibro and Addison's go, but my back was not doing good at all. Really bad pain with bending and really, any movement. I thought the surgery was going to make me better, but so far, I am not happy with all this pain still.

9:30am- PB toast
1pm- almond joy cookies (3)
6:30pm- chips and hummus, almond joy cookies
3 bottles of water

December 17, 2017

Super exhausted all day. I have a bruise or something on my elbow from having it on a chair last night. I just really want to sleep. Took 1 doxepin and 2 melatonin, so here's hoping.

9:30am- PB toast
11:30am- kiwi, banana, strawberries, grapes, raspberries
2:30pm- 5 almond joy cookies
6pm- edamame
2 bottles of water

December 18, 2017

Was hoping to sleep in, but that didn't happen. At least I was able to get some decent sleep, but still super exhausted. Hard to keep my eyes open all day, but got things done, cleaned kitchen, brought in wood, and vacuumed. Hurt my body, but who else is gonna do what needs to be done? Feeling super stressed today. More feeling of just wanting to get out of the situation/marriage and wondering if putting my body through work and raising my son's alone will make it worse than staying and trying to work whatever this is out.

9am- PB toast
12pm- shrimp
Ate too many cookies today
4 bottles of water

December 19, 2017

Stressing so much already and the day has just begun. Went to therapy and had a good session. Talked about how to start the new year and what to do about my husband and I.

My body is hating me and just wants to rest, but I am pushing too much, and I feel a crash coming. Need help and I'm just not getting it. I want to escape. Why can't my husband see the pain I am in and just pitch in to help and make my life easier?

8:30am- PB toast
6pm- rice, veggies and tilapia
3 bottles of water

December 20, 2017

My body is really feeling the stress from everything. I'm so tired and just need some sleep. Oh, and a vacation.

9:30am- PB toast
6pm- grits
10:15pm- edamame
2 bottle of water

December 21, 2017

Super exhausted. Laid around all day. Just so worn down and exhausted. Took 2 doxepin and 2 melatonin so I can sleep tonight and tomorrow. So mad I had to miss my oldest son's game but there was no way I would have made it safely down. My body is a mess. Did ACV 3 times today. I think it helped, not sure, but I'll keep doing it to see. I've read that it helps with energy and it's really good for you, so we shall see if it does anything.

9:30am- PB toast
6pm- sushi
3 bottles of water

December 22, 2017

Slept for 10 hours and rested in bed til 12:30pm. Did ACV twice. I think it's working but could be a placebo thing.
Super depressed today, and it showed because my youngest noticed it and asked why I was so sad. Had a talk with my husband, not sure where that is gonna end up. I'm just so exhausted with everything. I really need a pick me up. I can't be everything and everywhere for everyone. I don't want to fail

at writing like I failed at massage (not that I failed, I just had to quit because my body failed).

I need to have something of my own, so I feel I have a purpose besides just being a mom. They won't need me forever.

Hopefully I won't get worse health wise. I feel like in the last year I have gone downhill so fast.

I applied for disability today, so hopefully that will be something that will work out for me. We shall see.

12:30pm- PB toast
6pm- big mac and fries
To many coconut almond cookies
4 bottles of water

December 23, 2017

Woke up with some energy. Slept 6 hours-but tossed and turned a lot. Energy went away pretty quickly after going out in public. Got my nose ring changed out. Went to the mall and *Target*. When I got home I felt like I could have napped and should have. Did a 40 min yoga session. I'm so ready for bed now.

8:30am- PB toast
4pm- chips and almond joy cookies
83:0pm- bowl of *Lucky Charms*
2 bottles of water

December 24, 2017

Hurt my back somehow (cleaning the house) and couldn't stand up. Tried to take it easy but my back hurt pretty bad all night.

8:40am- PB toast
Almond joy cookies
6pm- rice, shrimp, carrots, Brussel sprouts
2 bottles of water

December 25, 2017

Slept crappy. Having body pain/back pain, especially when I would try to bend over.

9am- PB toast
3pm- salads (quinoa, carrots, and Brussel sprouts)
4 bottles of water

December 26, 2017

Slept for 6 hours. Felt ok, but a bit tired.
Cleaned up the kitchen, vacuumed, and put all the Christmas decorations away. My body didn't like that at all.

PB toast
Quinoa salad
Popcorn
Spaghetti
PB toast
5 bottles of water

December 27, 2017

I got 1 hour of sleep between 3-5am, 20 min between 8-8:45am, and a 15 min nap, because Haelee needed to bark at every sound she heard. Today has been a horrible struggle. My mid back is hurting (like a rib is out of place). I need to get that looked at.
I just need some sleep. Took 1 doxepin at 5:30pm and another one at 7pm to help with sleep.

PB toast
4 tacos
Popcorn
Coconut ice cream
2 bottles of water

December 28, 2017

Got 10 hours of sleep total (I think I got 6 hours straight). Didn't get out of bed til 12:30pm. Felt great to sleep. I could have gotten in a good nap if my youngest was quieter, but I got what I could, and even though I could have taken another nap, I felt pretty good.

Did 30 min of elliptical, 10 min of mat work, and 40 min yoga (restorative)- to help with the low back and hips.

PB toast
Banana
Chips
PB toast
Chips
4 bottles of water

December 29, 2017

Took us 7 hours of driving, but we made it down to my dad's. My body was in so much pain (it started about ½ way into the drive). Hopefully it won't be bad in the morning.

PB toast
Roasted veggies at *Applebee's*
BBQ ribs
3 bottles of water

December 30, 2017

Got up and got ready to go out and visit everyone. Didn't sleep great, but the bed was so comfy. My body hates me for putting it through that drive. It was so great seeing everyone and I loved how the boys just bonded quickly and loved meeting my side of the family. Wish we could have stayed longer, but I definitely want to go back soon. The drive home only took 4.5 hours and that was with stopping to pee and then getting gas.
Exhausted and in a whole lot of pain, but we made it home and now I get to crawl into my own bed. Let's hope for some healing sleep.

Oatmeal and toast
French fries
Salad and veggies

December 31, 2017

Pain level is a 7. Headache and so exhausted. Despite that, I took the boys to see *Jumanji- Welcome to the Jungle*. I came home and slept.
I hate having to miss out on hanging out with friends, it sucks so bad. I just want to be out having fun, not being sick and in pain.
Threw up- I think from the pain and headache. I was glad that I got to ring in the new year with my boys though. Goodbye 2017- Hello to a healing 2018

Oatmeal and toast
Movie theater popcorn

January 1, 2018

Happy new year! I love being able to start the new year with my boys. Even though we had to miss out on the party at our friend's house, I am so happy it was just us.
After resting all day yesterday. I felt about 70% recovered. I was able to get in a workout, laundry, and made dinner. It was good to have some energy back. I feel like I still could have taken a rest day today, but I could also tell my body needed to get some movement or the pain from not getting blood moving through my muscles was going to start affecting me.
I enjoyed being up and talking with the boys. It was/is their last full day here, so I wanted to be present.
Trying to come into the new year positive but I was really upset that I had to miss out on time with friends and that my husband got to enjoy it. I want him to have fun and I'm not mad at him, just upset that he can still do things, which he should be able to do. I was hoping that he would have come home to be with us for the ball drop but I'm also glad he stayed and enjoyed himself. Trying to not be resentful (I had to work hard on that today). Having to miss things because my body hates me is so hard to deal with and it just seems to keep getting worse.

January 2, 2018

Even though I only got 3 hours and 40 min of sleep. I woke up at 5am feeling like I got rest. Today was uneventful, which was nice. Sometimes those are the best days after getting shitty sleep.

Rested the rest of the evening.

Was able to juice today, I've really missed having that. I need to get back to eating better/more too. It's been hard with being so tired and in pain. All I want to do is rest. The last thing I want to do is put effort into cooking. Even with meal planning, if I don't have the energy, it's not going to get done.

January 3, 2018

Got 9 hours and 50 min of sleep. Taking 2 doxepin helped with that. Didn't wake up feeling overly exhausted like I normally would after taking it. Was hoping to start the day earlier, but I want to make sure I'm not pushing my body. Learning to let it rest as much as it needs.

Other than the struggle with homeschooling today, I think I sort of got some things done. Trying not to stress, so just letting things happen and work themselves into a flow is all I can really do.

My body did good today, hardly noticed the low back pain- only with certain movements. I need to get into the chiro and schedule a massage to help things feel better. I was about a level 2 whole body pain.

I hit my hand on the corner of the table and it hurt all the way to my shoulder. I couldn't grip or close the hand and it took over an hour for the pain to stop. Realizing how slow my body heals is sad. The little things that shouldn't hurt can really take me down.

I really need to just stick with the diet. There are so many alternatives, I just need to do it. I hate going out for things though, so it makes it hard. All I can do is just do better tomorrow, right?

January 4, 2018

I was hoping for a better day. Lost ALL my stuff on my laptop. Everything was gone when I did the update. Looked on our desk top computer and everything I transferred from my laptop to there is gone. It was like being punched in the stomach. Went over to see if my friend's husband could fix it and he couldn't find anything, so he finished wiping it and he installed *Dropbox*, so this wouldn't happen again. When I got home I was trying to reinstall windows (office) and couldn't find it, so I opened up "my office" and I saw all my documents. Sitting here now trying to save them, but office is refusing to finish it's install. Trying to stay positive that it will work. When I went to do my workout, I just wasn't in it, but made myself and I pushed past the 20 min and did 32 min on the elliptical while I read. I really just want today to be over and tomorrow to be a really good day.

Today's stress was awful. My body was super pissed, and I could feel the effect of it.

January 5, 2018

Woke up feeling hopeful and ready to get things loaded on my laptop, but it had other plans. It has completely stopped working properly. I learned that I did not purchase a protection plan for it, so I am just stuck with it. I have chosen to just let it go, don't let it affect me negatively anymore and I have moved on. I got all I was planning to put on the laptop loaded onto my desktop. I will have to work from that until I am able to buy another (better) laptop. Moving forward so I can start writing again.

I had a Dr. appointment today. Got some cupping and acupuncture done. I really needed both. It was a 2 ½ hour appointment.

There were a few things I really wanted to get done today, but I will just keep adjusting things as needed until I can catch up from falling behind.

I hardly ate anything today and felt really exhausted. Pain wasn't too bad, but I know I needed to stress dose. I was disappointed that I was unable to get a workout in. God knows I needed the stress relief.

My boys keep me motivated to stay positive, fight daily, and keep calm in stressful situations. Teaching them to not overreact, stay calm, and stay focused on the ultimate goal is what I want them to see coming from me. I want them to know their mom is a fighter and that it will inspire them to fight for things as well.

Hoping tomorrow is full of positive energy and that we can just enjoy the day.

January 6, 2018

Only got 2 hours and 40 min of sleep. Computer reboot and stress of it had me up way more than I wanted, but it worked, so I am happy about that. We shall see if it works for a longer period of time. I now know to save on different programs to ensure the safety of my documents. Got all the things loaded, saved, and signed in. The number of things I lost was heartbreaking. Letters to my boys, books I started, poems, pictures, and a mess of other things.

My body is in so much pain, I need a good night's sleep to heal. Apparently, I am not able to let go of losing so much from the laptop. It still makes me sick thinking about it.

January 7, 2018

I knew I was going to either be hurting really bad or exhausted today. Pain was only about a 3, but I could feel every move in my low back. It was pretty bad, it might be the reasons my hips were hurting. I slept til 10am but didn't get good sleep.

Didn't get all the things I wanted done, but I was trying to listen to my body. I really need to start eating more. I've been slacking again. That could be affecting how I feel too.

I'm so exhausted and ready for bed. Ready to start my week off right.

January 8, 2018

Took 2 doxepin last night to help me get some rest. I got 8 hours and 50 min of motionless good sleep. I wish my restless would be deep sleep, that was 2 hours and 10 min. If back pain and noise would just go away. Maybe I should invest in some ear plugs.

Went to the chiro and I have c3-c4 out of place as well as a rib. I want to try to get a massage this week as well.

My back seems to be having more bad days and every time I do flexion, it hurts. Bending down isn't bad, it's coming up or after I carry something more the 5lbs, it hurts. Hoping chiro will help. I see the surgeon on Feb. 1st, so we will see what he says. I'm so tired of my body hurting and I hate mentioning it because it just sounds like I'm whining all the time about pain.

January 9, 2018

Fell asleep pretty quickly last night. Slept ok til I heard a crash at 5:20am. Got out of bed to see what it was. Stupid shower thing fell in the tub. Took me a while to get back to sleep but got in about an hour and a half. Therapy was good. Talked mostly about the laptop issue and *Hero's and Villain's* and how I should use that time to write and de-stress and just enjoy some "me time" without feeling guilty.

One thing I learned about myself last year is that my body is weak. The more I push it and force it to do things it can't and shouldn't, it pushes back and causes horrible pain and flare-ups. This year I am going to listen to it more, so it won't destroy me. I've already missed out on things I've wanted to do, but listened to my body, rested, and it sucked, but it was what my body needed.

January 10, 2018

Slept horrible last night. Woke up thinking someone was in the house. Thought I heard someone come in through the spider room door. I need to lock it for peace of mind. I know if someone was in the house, Haelee would have barked. Still, I was a bit shaken. Had a hard time falling back asleep. Woke up again a couple hours later with heart palpitations. I don't know what was going on.

Struggled to get up for my chiro appointment, but I made it. Felt good to have an adjustment.

January 11, 2018

Took 2 doxepin last night and slept pretty good. Got in 7 hours and 20 min with 1 hour and 47 min of tossing and turning. I felt rested when I woke up. Felt like I needed to go back to bed after being up for an hour though. When my husband was leaving for work, he discovered our van was broken into and his power tools were gone. I really hate this neighborhood. I wish the druggie neighbors were gone. Would be so nice to be out in the country where this doesn't happen. I would love to catch someone stealing from us. Especially with my gun. Not to kill them, but to make sure they think twice about stealing from someone again. Maybe a sign in our window saying, "the first shot is a warning, the 2nd is your funeral." Hopefully our landlord will get the flood lights and security up and working soon.

Got to actually make dinner tonight. I made panko crusted tofu and rice. Feels like forever since I've had the energy to actually cook something. The one thing I like about being 'vegan-ish" is the ease of making things. So much easier on me when I do actually cook.

January 12, 2018

I tossed and turned all night. Probably my excitement for today.

The drive was nice- listened to *Gone With the Wind* on *Audible*. Got into Portland at 2pm. The drive was good; no traffic. My body did ok. Got to my room and unpacked, then sat and read some. Peace and quiet…. It was so nice.

Resting up for tomorrow. It's going to be a long day, but I am so excited that I get to meet Stephen Amell!!

January 13, 2018

Didn't sleep great last night and when my alarm went off, I didn't want to get up. I looked at my phone and saw a FB notification that Stephen Amell liked my blog post. That woke me up. I was so happy, it was a perfect start to the day. It made getting up and ready easier. Got to the convention and grabbed a wheelchair. My right side of my low back was hurting with every step. The wheelchair helped, but I was still in a lot of pain. I also learned that having a wheelchair gets you in the front of every line. It was better than the platinum VIP pass.

Did a couple panels, which I got to see Stephen Amell (got a little choked up seeing him, but saw him a lot throughout the day, so that helped me not lose it when I met him). He's just as amazing as I had him built up in my head.

David Ramsey was a big surprise. Such an amazing nice guy. Got to talk to him for a while about L5-S1 fusion. It was pretty cool.

Josh Sagarra kissed my cheek. It was surprising. I wasn't impressed with Emily or Katie. They were the least friendliest celebs there.

I'm in so much pain and so exhausted. My body is saying no more, don't make me do this again…. Just 1 more day.

January 14, 2018

I tossed and turned all night. Could not get comfortable. My back was so bad. I just had to get through 1 panel and then a 3-hour long drive home. I walked about ½ mile to the convention center, sat for the panel, walked back and drove home. The drive was great- it went fast, but I could slowly feel my back getting worse.

My body was not happy. Hips, legs, LB, were all just screaming. It was difficult to walk around. I managed to get the bare minimum done, but I just have to be ok with that.

January 15, 2018

Slept pretty decent last night. I was able to sleep for 2 hours straight.

Got to go to the chiro and get adjusted. He thinks maybe my low back muscles have atrophied so that's why I'm in so much pain all the time, but with having Addison's and Fibro, it could be my body just not working right and not healing properly because of the stress.

So, I'll do core and LB strengthening to hit those deeper muscles and see. He's still waiting on notes from the surgeon, so he can start adjusting my LB more intensely. It needs something. I also need to get a massage, my body is really needing that.

I'm exhausted, my body is hurting so bad. I'm glad I am resting this week. I think it's a good idea to take a week from traveling and just rest. I hate having to rest because it makes me miss things that I want to be at, but my body needs to recover. But how much does it really help? I honestly don't know because I never give my body the time to rest.

January 16, 2018

Slept pretty shitty last night. I was up at 6am and couldn't go back to sleep- not for lack of trying. I got out of bed at 8am.

I did a 30 min leg workout, didn't think I would make it, but I did and then I wanted to make sure I got in all my steps. So, I jumped on the elliptical for 25 mins. My hips are hurting a bit, but it's a good sore…. I hope.

Made dinner again tonight, even though I was exhausted.

January 17, 2018

Thought I would sleep better taking doxepin and smoking, but I fell asleep fast and was tossing all night. Got in a good little chunk from about 5:45-7:20am. I wish I could get a good 4 hours in. Had a chiro appointment at 9am-I hate being up and out of the house that early, it's so hard. Felt great to get adjusted, I can start to feel a difference, especially in my neck. The low back workouts are helping a bit, so I'll continue to see how that goes. Had an eye dr. appointment today. I have a stigmatism in both eyes. L eye is worse and by my next visit I'll probably have to have a special contact for that eye. He gave me different contacts to try. Not sure if it was from being dilated or if the contacts just aren't strong enough, but my vision was blurry the rest of the day.

Noticed a boil on my leg and bruises from my socks. My body hates me so much.

January 18, 2018

Shitty night's sleep-again. This was bad, too much awake time in between 3am-4:42am. It was almost like I had a burst of energy. It took me a while to fall back asleep.

I went and got my hair cut today. Decided to stay short, went a tad bit shorter this time and more layered in the back- really love it. Not so much curly though. But still cute and easy to maintain.

Called to check on my disability and to see if they were receiving everything. D.D. was no help- the lady was rude and then transferred me to my case worker- who never called back- maybe tomorrow. We shall see how that whole process goes.

Noticed that boil thing came back and now it's red. I should have just left it alone. I will keep an eye on it, just in case.

Time for bed.

January 20, 2018

So yesterday was…interesting. Horrible pain in my hips woke me up, then my calf cramped.

I went and got spray paint and painted the coffee table… Then lost all function in my right hand from spraying. It hurt and ached. I couldn't grip anything. Tried writing 10 hours later and couldn't. 10 min of spraying shouldn't affect me, but I also have an already weak grip and failing body. Later on, after it had dried, I went to move the table to the porch and tripped, hitting my shin on it. I should have just crawled back into bed. Having a hard time still and it's been almost 24 hours.

Didn't sleep good last night. Woke up around 12:30am and didn't fall back to sleep til around 2:45am. Then I tossed all night.

Tried to go for a walk and my back started to hurt really bad- about 3 blocks into it, but I was hoping it would get better. I honestly don't know how I function most days. God gives me enough- sometimes I feel like I'm not even in my body and just watching it move.

My body hurts so bad.

Was stocking the fire and my back froze up. Couldn't stand. My whole body is so achy. Took doxepin and melatonin- gonna smoke and then pass out and hopefully sleep.

I wish people would be more understanding of those with chronic pain/invisible illness. It's not easy, but they sure like to judge.

January 21, 2018

Slept til 11:30am. Got some good rest but feeling exhausted all day.

Did not get close to getting my goals met, but that's ok. I got laundry done and that was the important one.

My body could have slept all day. Today was uneventful since I did nothing but rest.

January 22, 2018

Tried the ear plugs last night and I think I need a couple more nights with them to see. It was nice not being woke up by all the small noises, but I still tossed and turned. Mainly because my back hurt and then around 4-5am the plugs started to hurt my ears.

I went to the chiro, *Central Market*, *Whole Foods*, *Silver Safari*- it was a lot, but I made it through it. Felt like I had the energy, but the pain was not good. My back just isn't letting up, but I'm glad my arms and hands feel better. Still can't grip like before, but the pain from spray painting has gotten better.

Got most of the errands and stuff done today- minus the cleaning one- but that can be done another day.

I'm a little wound up, hopefully I can get to sleep.

January 24, 2018

Yesterday was a blur. Went to therapy. Drove down for the boy's game. The drive was awful. My body was hurting.

Today, I ran around for a bit, got wine bottles, looked for books, looked for lamps at *Goodwill*. Read, wrote, relaxed. My body really needed to just stay in bed, but I didn't. Gonna try to stay down a bit more tomorrow.

So exhausted and in pain tonight. Just want to crawl in bed and sleep for a few days. Ear plugs help, but they hurt my ears too much to continue to try.

January 25, 2018

My sleep chunks are bigger with wearing the ear plugs, but I have to take them out because they start to hurt. Wonder if I didn't sleep on my side, and just stayed on my back, if that would make a difference?

Woke up this morning at about 5:30am and couldn't go back to sleep til around 7am. Then back up at 8am.

Went to the chiro, not sure if it was the adjustment or the workout, but my back and hips were in so much pain tonight, it was really difficult to move around.

One thing that frightens me is failing my boys... in any way. I want to be here for them, but my body doesn't allow it most of the time. I want them to know that I tried to do my best- all the time- that I sacrificed so much time, money, health, etc. to be there for everything I could, even when it caused me so much pain. I hope they know this.

January 26, 2018

My sleep chunks were good. The new ear plugs were less painful. I still only got about 5 hours and I was so exhausted.

I got up and cleaned out and vacuumed the car and van. Picked up all the trash from the yard and spider room. Vacuumed the house, got my youngest through his school work, read a book, went to *Target*, and worked out. It was like my body was going, but my mind was in slow motion. Everything hurt so bad, but I needed to get it done.

January 28, 2018

Yesterday I started to have an adrenal crisis. I pushed myself to hard the last couple days when I knew my body was feeling weak. So I went to pick up Silverbiotics and then I was going to go to go grab some groceries. I felt dizzy and more nauseous on the way. It was like cars that passed me were a blur and my vision itself was blurry. Felt like I was going to faint. Decided it was best not to try and get groceries so I just went home and rested.

Lost strength in my legs- I could barely walk- everything hurt so bad. Low BP-higher resting heart rate. Mild crisis. Glad my husband came home from his gaming night to make sure I was ok. It's always so scary to go through that, especially alone or with the boys. I hate that they have to see me like that. I really hate this disease.

Today was better. Stress dosing really helps, but it still has me down. Taking cold meds just to boost my immune system and give my body some help fighting whatever is trying to take me out.

Can't wait til Friday to see Dr. K. need to call my endocrinologist- something just hasn't felt right for a while, and I need to be cautious because who knows what my body might be developing.

Also, being able to finally see my surgeon about my low back. It seems to be getting worse. Not like before; isolated to the L. SI joint but should not be this painful.

I feel like I just keep getting worse and no matter what I do to help- it fails. My husband shouldn't have to live this life with me. He suffers from it and it's hard to watch and disappoint him so much. I'm so moody all the time because I'm in so much pain constantly. Everything annoys me. When I do have a good day, it doesn't seem to last long.

Going from a level 7 pain to a level 3 pain is huge and I am easier to deal with on those days. But they are few.

I know it's dramatic and stupid to say but when I have these stupid crisis, I feel like I'm dying, and it will be the last time I'll see the boys, my husband, or anyone. It's like death is right there just waiting.

I felt I missed out on the whole weekend with the boys and it sucks, I hate that they had to see me in such pain. Next time I'll be better. I hate Addisons…..... and fibro. Though this was 95% Addisons.

January 29, 2018

Another day to recover. Feeling about 60% better.

Went in for a massage. She was ok, not great, but it was better than not having one. Expected more from someone who had been doing it for 13 years.

The chiro is sending in the letter he wrote to disability. Really appreciate that he is behind me on this.

One thing I will also do is keep fighting and show my boys that you don't give up just because something tries to bring you down.

January 30, 2018

Didn't sleep great last night. Ear plugs may work, but my husband still moves a lot which is disrupting my sleep. Not sure if we will ever be able to co-sleep. I really need good sleep too, but not sure he'll want to stay in a sexless/separate bed type of marriage.

I feel there is more wrong with me and that's why I don't seem to get better. Lots of people on the groups I'm in struggle so much daily-would be nice to hear more about how their marriages work instead of just the aches, pains, and Dr. complaints.

Had a good therapy session. Talked about the age gap with my husband and I and how some of his temperament, and "forgetfulness" could be ADHD. Which he was not in any type of agreeance with. He was kind of moody too. Not really hearing what I was trying to say but twisting it, so it made me sound like I was saying he did nothing. So frustrating. That's why I'd rather just message him. He gets too upset, too fast, and doesn't listen or hear what I'm trying to say. I guess we just push it aside with all the other problems that never get resolved. I guess if we can just be happy with where we are and never fix anything- we can grow old and resent our lives- living for the boys and potential grand kids. At this point- it's hard to say where I'm at. I'm just trying to keep my sanity with homeschooling, author stuff, the boys, my friends, house stuff, and life. Trying to fit him in when we are so far apart is hard.

My body is still trying to recover. Today it was weak and painful to walk. Felt like my shins were trying to rip through my skin. I was walking, and my muscles totally gave out. It's like they didn't want me walking. My joints all over were really achy and my forearms felt like they were going to explode. I know I should be resting and not doing anything, but my oldest has his Senior night that I don't want to miss out on. Just don't know what my body is going to do.

February 1, 2018

Yesterday we drove down for my oldest son's last home basketball game. He did so amazing, played like he is ready for college ball. The other teams coach came up to us after the game and said he was hard to guard and that he did a great job and gave his team a run for their money.

My body was in so much pain. Got to talk with an old friend at the game and she recommended a couple books for me to read (*Food Over Medicine* and *How Not to Die*). I'm excited to start reading those.

Today was pretty painful and I'm so exhausted. Went to see my surgeon today and he doesn't know why I'm in so much pain. He says I shouldn't be, so we are going to start with some PT to see how that goes. Something has to work.

I'm trying everything I can so I can have a "normal" active life. I want to work again. Writing is a hobby that might never bring in any money.

My husband is again stressed over money and made me feel horrible today because I "take all the money" he makes. I need to find a way to support me and the boys. I want to be independent and not feel weird about spending money on just normal things (food, dr. appt. etc.). Especially since we can't figure out our relationship-I'm gonna need a way to live on my own and support the kids. I can't do that if I'm always feeling how I do. So exhausted and in pain. I need a caregiver.

February 2, 2018

Slept really bad. Woke up feeling worse.

Had my appointment with Dr. K. I finally told her how I have been feeling the past few days, and how I just can't seem to kick it. My urine sample came back showing I was dehydrated (which is weird since I was drinking a ton of water). She said my body just wasn't pulling it in. She took some blood and put me on an IV drip. So exhausted and run down.

Struggled with getting to my PT appointment, but made it and did a light session. Hopefully I can get the back pain under control.

Worn down and tired of this autoimmune. I need good sleep this weekend.

February 4, 2018

Spent all day yesterday in bed recovering and all day today on the couch, recovering. Missed going to the Super bowl party. Yet another gathering I've missed due to the stupid Addisons.

I did manage to get some laundry done and cleaned the kitchen a bit. Which really exhausted me. Wish my husband would have jumped on that and got it done, but no surprise there. I hope I will feel better tomorrow. I need a good day.

Sleep hasn't been great-even with the ear plugs (but really when have I ever gotten good sleep). Gotta get that figured out.

Here's to a night of rest- hopefully.

February 5, 2018

For only getting 2 hours of sleep last night, I had a burst of energy today. I could not shut my mind down at all. So, I got up and wrote. Started a new book/journal for my journey down the autoimmune reversal.

Went to PT/Chiro and then little man's basketball practice. I'm exhausted now and it's 10pm. I made it through the day though. My body actually pulled me through on pretty much no sleep. Wonder how I'll feel tomorrow?

My brain feels like it's starting to shut down now, so maybe my body will stop hurting (cramps from being off BC). Cleaning out my body. It's gonna suck having a period again. Oh well, it's all for my health.

February 6th through March 27th, I wrote about my journey with the whole food plant-based diet. You can purchase that book on *Amazon* (Fighting Addison's Disease and Fibromyalgia: My 50-day journey on a WFPB diet)

FIGHTING MOM

I feel like I have been fighting for so long, that it has just become a battle that I might not win. Every time I try something new, I swear I get brand new symptoms or something weird happens to my body.

I love the diet change I made and that made a TON of the Fibromyalgia symptoms go away. I have strayed off the diet at times because life gets so hectic, kids graduate, lots of traveling, and other excuses. I am back to sticking to the vegan diet because in all honesty, it's what has worked for dealing with the fibro.

Now, Addisons has me on a whole other battlefield. This one I just can't get control of. If it's not figuring out the right dosage (yes I still have troubles with that), it's having a crisis, or avoiding sick people, trying not to stress over things, or not being able to function because I used all my spoons before 10am.

I am a mom and a wife. HOW THE FUCK DO I AVOID STRESS AND SICKNESS!?!?!?!

Journal Entry: March 2018- July 2018

<u>**March 28, 2018**</u>

Got up and got ready for a run. Slept really bad last night, but still felt ok. I made it 4.46 miles. My first mile was almost 10 min and my last was about 8.5 min. My times are looking better and it's getting easier.

This whole not working thing and helping out financially is really getting me depressed. I should just embrace that I can be at home and be able to see my kids. I do everything and try to be here for them. I have the time to write (which I don't put enough time into).

I feel so depressed I don't want too, but if I actually did it, I would probably do a lot better and feel better. Need to get out of this funk. I have nothing to complain about, yet here I am being a whiny bitch. UGH! Change my perspective, change my life.... I wish it were that simple. I really need to do it though. Stop complaining and just enjoy the blessed life I have. I really do love my babies and I have a pretty good life, but depression is no joke.

March 29, 2018
Allergies are not kind. Had a stress flare last night and one tonight. My body needs some really good sleep.
Was able to get in a little run today, painful, but got it in.

March 31, 2018
Having R side pain. Taking another rest day. Felt so crappy. No energy, high pain, feeling so drained and achy.
Every time the sun comes out I swear my body decides to get sick or be in a ton of pain.

April 2, 2018
No motivation, so I just lazed on the couch all day. Yes, I get that I need these days, but I still hate them.

April 5, 2018
I got a 4-hour chunk of sleep last night which was great.
Ran today, only 3 miles. My ankle was still hurting from the running shoes. Was glad I could exchange them yesterday and go back to the *Asics*.
My husband and I are going to try to go to one another's counseling sessions to see if that can help. I guess it's a step into a direction we are still unclear of.

April 8, 2018

My older 2 boys and I ran in a 10k race today. Boys did so amazing. They ran hard, and I am so proud of them.

My oldest: 1st place in age group- 9th overall- 7.09 m/mi

Middle guy: 3rd place in age group- 20th overall- 7.40m/mi

Me: 6th place in age group- 56th overall- 8.40m/mi

It was so much fun to be able to run this with them. Just to be able to run at all was amazing. Hopefully we can make this our annual thing.

Had to rest the rest of the day. My body was so exhausted. I took an hour nap, then got up and finished laundry and made dinner. The boys helped with cleaning the kitchen.

April 9, 2018

Went to my endo today. Really just wanted to sleep in and rest all day but can't miss appointments. She had blood drawn, checking me for clotting tracers and inflammation tracers, among other things. She wants me to do a bone density test to make sure the hydrocortisone hasn't started to make my bones weak yet, because that's just what my body would need.

Glad to see my husband helping with the house today, without being asked. The last thing I wanted to do today was laundry, so I was happy to see he got that done.

My youngest son's neck was bothering him, so I worked on his it a little bit. My hands couldn't do more than 5 min unfortunately. Sucks because I want to get back into massaging so bad. I have to stop dwelling on it and just move on. I can't even cut up vegetables without pain in my hands and forearms, massaging is just out of the question.

April 14, 2018

It's been a slow week. Taking off running may have been a bad idea. I feel grumpy but maybe it's the weather.

I wrote to the Congresswoman about being denied disability and heard back the next day from one of her reps, which was amazing. I really hope they can help me out. Praying hard that they can, and I can start figuring some things out.

April 17, 2018

Took me 2 days to recover from yard work. I hate being down. 1st day I couldn't walk, and it was so painful to stand. Had to use my wheelchair. Day 2, I was so exhausted and weak. I spent the day on the couch.

Finally got to run. Should not have taken a week off. My body definitely needs to exercise. I felt awful that whole week. I was only able to make it 2.5 miles before my legs just stopped, but it felt good. My back hurt a lot after but got better as the day went on.

Had our couples therapy session with my therapist today. It went ok. I really could have used one for myself, but it was a step for us. We shall see how everything pans out.

April 24, 2018

So much has happened in a week. Nothing really changed with my husband and I. He took off Friday to help clean for my oldest son's party, but he just played video games. I finally got up and cleaned, but I was in so much pain, it made me sick and I got to spend time vomiting instead of resting.

I was upset that we didn't get to have a good party for my son's 18th. I wanted it to be fun, but gaming messed that all up.

My back is bothering me and seems to get worse each day. I can't keep having all this pain and exhaustion. I'm done hurting all the time. Back surgery should have worked. I feel like that was just a waste of time and energy because the pain is still there.

My youngest had his 1st swim meet for Special Olympics. He did amazing but was disqualified because he swam faster than the time he was allowed to get. So frustrating. I hated seeing him upset. It's not fair to those athletes who work hard to PR (personal record) and then get DQ'd for it.

Got an email from the Senator's rep and then a phone call. Talking to the lady I learned that I'm pretty much getting denied disability because I'm not on a bunch of pain meds and narcotics, so insane. She said she has seen this so many times and it's sad and it needs to change.

Seems like one thing after another. I'm too tired to be dealing with this much stress.

May 1, 2018

Can't believe it's been so long since I've journaled. I had a pretty low-key week. I was so exhausted, I didn't get anything done.

Today I went for a 6.2-mile run, mowed the yard and went for a 10 min bike ride. Half way through mowing the backyard my inguinal muscle started to hurt so bad. My back had been hurting for a couple days but I wanted to do something, I can't just keep sitting around. I'm so tired of feeling like this. I just want the pain to stop.

The pain got so bad towards the evening that I couldn't walk.

May 8, 2018

The day I ran and mowed took a big toll on my body. Had to go see my surgeon on May 2nd. MRI on May 3rd. Got in to see the chiro on the 3rd and 4th. Was finally able to walk with minimal pain on the 4th. Went and saw the chiro again yesterday. Got a call from the surgeon's nurse today. MRI results show nothing new.

Going to have to stop running so my back will be able to heal properly. Seeing my chiro 3x has made the back a bit better. Wish insurance didn't limit the visits because they help so much. Running has really made the process slow down. I hate to have to give it up for now, but I can't be in this kind of pain all the time.

I feel like I keep spiraling into depression because I can't do anything. My stress has been off the charts and today with my husband losing his temper and breaking my youngest son's sword that his oldest brother got him- having to handle him being so upset about it- it really took a toll on me. My body hurts so bad that I couldn't sit still because it felt like every nerve in my body was freaking out. I wanted to scream and tear off my skin to make it stop. I can't seem to beat the depression. I stopped writing and editing, I can't focus or find joy in anything. I just want to be happy again. I want to write again. I have to stop letting this bring me down, but I also have no fight left. I've lost or feel like I just keep losing everything and I can't take it anymore. I need me time. I need to reflect on what's good and I need to break this darkness. The pain and stress need to stop. I have to bring myself back, because I hate this person I am right now. She is killing me.

May 14, 2018

It was a rough weekend- ate off the diet and got sick and was in pain, but still was able to enjoy Mother's Day with my boys.

Took the boys to a trampoline park and almost shit my pants. Would have been so embarrassing, but I barely made it to the bathroom. My fault for not sticking with the diet.

I haven't done any writing or editing in a week now. I have to get back on track. I keep procrastinating, but things around the house need to be done.

May 22, 2018

I keep slacking on journaling.

More symptoms have been getting worse (the ones I keep ignoring), so today I will go in and see the neurologist to see about testing for MS and Lyme's. Would be nice to have some answers to why I feel so crappy and why things are getting worse.

I've been so depressed that I feel it's gotten out of hand and has affected my activity and life. I just want to do things, but also being in pain prevents me.

Couple days ago, I went in and got acupuncture and cupping done…. that sent me into a flare for a couple days. It was so bad.

I get to go home this weekend for Community Days. So happy that the boys (minus my oldest) will be coming with me.

June 1, 2018

I was pretty much bed ridden for 3 days after going home for Community Days. I wasn't supposed to be running but decided to do the 5K run…. and then there was basketball. Took my body a week to fully recover.

I really hate my diseases. I didn't let it stop me from having fun, but it sure put me down after.

Also found out that the MRI actually showed that I had a slight bulge and fissure on my R. side. Why did the surgeon not think this was "anything?" It obviously is affecting me, so it means something.

June 13, 2018

The craziness has subsided. Graduation festivities are done. I can't believe my baby boy is done and going to be on his own. I'm excited/scared for him, but I know he will do amazing things.

Got to have my dad visit for 5 days. It was nice having him here to help. My body held up ok through the stress of getting everything done, but I am exhausted still. I took a LOT of ibuprofen to get through it. It helped some but wish I had more energy and less pain. Summer has officially begun, and I am looking forward to some down time and nice weather.

June 15, 2018

Today was a bad day. So much pain, fatigue, and dizziness. I woke up and my hands were swollen, I was dizzy, my muscles felt so weak, shortness of breath, and pain. I spent the day on the couch. I was able to go get my hair trimmed, but it was a struggle to get there. I probably shouldn't have been driving.

Having a hard time focusing my eyes just to write this.

I'm wondering if my body is trying to detox the food I ate (and shouldn't have eaten). Maybe I should do a cleanse to help. I feel like shit. I'm tired of feeling like this.

On a good note, one of the Addison groups on Instagram wants to help promote my book. That's exciting.

June 16, 2018

Today I am 38! Had my lashes done, my youngest took me out for sushi, and we went for a walk (that I almost collapsed on). Not sure what is happening but my body the last few days has been horrible. Nausea, headaches, dizziness, shortness of breath, weak muscles, exhaustion and pain. UGH!

Even though it wasn't a "great" bday with a party and friends, I enjoyed the time I had to relax, finish a book and have some quality time with my little guy. My body wouldn't have been able to handle anything other than what it did today. That was a struggle in itself.

My body decided to say happy bday to me with a 3 day early start to my period. YAY for 38! I find it funny that in the 24 years I have had a period, this was the first time it has ever started on my birthday…. Interesting.

June 25, 2018

Friday, I left for Wenatchee to go to the *Kings of Leon* concert with my best friend/sister at the *Gorge*. I love going there. It's such a breathtaking view. I was feeling tired and run down, but excited.

Stopped by and got to see my niece for the first time. She is already 10 months old.

We went out to eat and about 20 min later, my stomach was so bloated, and I felt like I was going to vomit. Luckily, I didn't, but it was not fun.

My body didn't' like the cold (once the sun went down, it got really chilly) or sitting on the ground. I was in so much pain by the time the concert got done. Driving home was hell. It was dark, and I can't see in the dark. It started raining and I couldn't see the lines in the road. It was a scary drive home.

The next 2 days I was in so much pain. Saturday stayed in bed all day. I could barely walk. I wanted to get my nails done though, so I had my husband take me. Getting the foot scrub done was torture. I was tearing up because the pain was too much. The poor lady giving me the pedicure was sweet about it. The girl who did my manicure had my nails all crooked, she kept burning me with the machine that files off the shellac. I had to file my nails down, so they looked even before I let her paint them. I won't go back there. Came home and got back into bed.

Sunday was a little better but stayed on the couch and wrote.

I haven't been sleeping well, but what else is new.

Today I had therapy, chiro and had to take Haelee to the vet. My body wanted to stay in bed. I haven't been able to eat without feeling really sick. I get really nauseous, extremely bloated, and horrible pain every time I eat something. Got some meal replacement shakes to see if that will help. I can't not eat. My body just feels weaker everyday- no matter what I do, I just can't win.

June 30, 2018

My eating hasn't gotten any better. I have such horrible stomach pain when I eat anything. I smoked to see if that would help enough for me to eat. It did a little, but I also don't want to have to smoke every time I eat. Drinking the meal replacement shake is better, but I still feel so nauseous and still have the bloating.

Yesterday I went to the Endo and she is referring me to see a gastroenterologist. She had similar stomach issues in April and May, so she was sympathetic. I told her all the symptoms that I have been having and she thinks that is sounds like MS or Lyme's as well. She said my last blood work back in April showed I was low in protien and borderline with the potassium. Why is it so hard to get all these levels right? She did more blood work, so we shall see. I can't imagine it will look good since I haven't been able to really eat for like a week.

My shoulder is still not healed from when it started hurting on June 5th. Yesterday I went in for PT and Chiro and today I can barely lift my arm or move it around much because of the pain. The chiro said if it's not any better by next week he is going to order an MRI to be done, just in case. Why does my body fucking hate me so much?

I took my first TRX class (heavily modified). I wasn't able to do much in the class, thanks to my arm hurting, but I did get a feel for how the class is and how amazing the workout could be. I also was on the treadmill and my L. leg just gave out on me. I was lucky to catch myself and not fall off. Had that been the case, I would have cancelled our membership and never returned.

My husband and I are trying to figure out if we want a marriage or just a friendship. It is hard because I don't have any desire to have sex. It's been 8 months for us. We decided to try it the other night. I had to get high, so my body would be ok with being touched. I felt numb though. Some things that used to feel good, I couldn't even feel at all (could have been from being high). It was painful and not that enjoyable. Especially after, when the pain really set in. I hate to have him stay with me if I can't do one of the most basic wife things. I feel sad for our relationship, but also know that if we are to separate, we will remain good friends and do great co-parenting. I feel that he shouldn't have to stay with me to take care of me and not have any benefit from having a marriage. It's more like a caregiver/roommate situation and that isn't good for anyone.

July 1, 2018

Still having the stomach pains and extreme bloating after I eat anything. Even with the meal replacement shakes too. I think those are causing me to have some major gas as well. I hate being in so much pain, especially with eating.

I did manage to drag my ass to the gym. I needed to get out of the house and get my body moving. I wanted to just sleep all day, but I know that is not good for my body. I tried Excedrin PM last night to see if that would help with sleep. I didn't notice a difference. Should have just bought the trial pack.

I can't wait to get the sleep patch thing I ordered (damn Instagram ads). I hope those work. There is a 365-day guarantee on them, so if they don't work, I can always get my money back.

July 4, 2018

Well, today is the 4th of July. Happy Independence Day!! This is one of my favorite holidays. It's hot out, the kids all play in the water, adults are having fun, hanging out in the sun, drinking, BBQ-ing, and everyone is just happy. Since my stomach has had so many issues and I haven't been able to get into the gastroenterologist to figure out why, (I can't eat anything without having extreme bloating, nausea, and horrible stomach pain) I took matters into my own hands yesterday. I know that the gastroenterologist is going to want to do a colonoscopy... I'm not 100% ok with them sticking a scope up my ass and looking around. I know they will make me drink something that would cause me to have the fast potties and if they don't find anything, then I would be violated for nothing... but cleaned out. So, I went to the store and got some Exlax. Yesterday and today I have done Exlax and water. HOLY SHIT (pun intended). Literally peeing shit all the time. It's ok, because tomorrow I will start with just having the vegan shakes. If I can do ok on those, then the next day I will try out some food to see if it worked. I really hope it does, because I really want to enjoy food again.

Had a blast watching all the kids (and husbands) enjoy the fireworks. No one was blown up or hurt, so that was a plus.

Very exhausting day. Especially since the 2 days before I had only gotten 2.5 hours one night and 3 the next.

July 5, 2018

Today didn't turn out how I wanted it at all. I woke up and my legs were really weak. I had my shake. I still had some nausea with it, but the bloating wasn't there, so that was a plus. I got really winded walking from the couch to the dining room (maybe 10 steps). I was out of breath. Came back to lay down on the couch and was even more out of breath. I was having a hard time. It felt like my body had just been through a 10-mile hard run. I had my son grab the wheelchair, because I knew I wouldn't be able to walk without difficulty.

Wheeled around and was starting a grocery list and had to lay down on the floor because I was starting to get really dizzy.

After laying there for about 20-30 min, I got into the wheelchair and as my husband was wheeling me to the couch, it got really hard to breath. I just couldn't slow my breathing down no matter what. I said something is wrong and leaned forward and I was on the ground trying to get some air into my lungs. Tears were streaming down my face. My oldest son was trying to get me to calm down and take deep breaths; steady my breathing. Even though I really wanted too, I couldn't do it. My middle son rushed my youngest to the bedroom and stayed in there, keeping him calm and distracted.

My husband called 911 and they were here within 3 min (so thankful they have a station that is so close). My son and husband kept telling them that I needed my injection, but they hadn't heard of Addison's Disease and it wasn't a drug that they carried. My son and husband were very adamant about it, telling them if I don't get it I could die. My injection kit was apparently expired, so they were not going to administer it. And the Dr. they called at the ER told them not to give it to me. I was rushed to the hospital.

At the hospital they thought it could be a panic attack, anxiety, or heart attack. Of course, I can barely talk. Even though I had slowed my breathing down, it was still extreme. The Dr. refused to give me Hydrocortisone, he said he would call my Endo and talk with her. He came back and told the nurse to give me something to help slow my breathing. Before they left I told the nurse I had to pee. I couldn't use my legs at all, they just wouldn't support my body, so they gave me a bed pan. It hurt so bad to go. It was like something was blocking the pee from getting out and it was awful.

Finally, I was able to go after about 5 min of trying and the first 30 plus seconds was so painful.

The nurse came in to give me the meds that would slow my breathing. I had told her that my arms and legs felt like they were filling up with blood and going to explode. She said ok and then cleared the line with saline and then put in the meds. In about 3 seconds all my muscles tightened and tensed up and started to pull me into a ball, I couldn't breathe at all, like I couldn't even get air into the back of my throat.

I was shaking, and my muscles were no longer in my control. I started to fade out and even though she was telling me to calm down and breathe, it sounded like she was far away from me, everything went black, and then I was able to start breathing and getting more air.

I was hit with exhaustion, but I wasn't struggling to breathe now. Once my body relaxed a bit and I was laying down and almost falling asleep, I completely stopped breathing. The nurse was yelling at me and started pounding on my chest so I would start breathing, but I wasn't responding. I could hear her, but she sounded very far away, she kept hitting my chest and yelling, but I was slipping away. She threw an oxygen tube on me and hit me some more in the chest trying to force me to take in a deep breath. Finally, I was able to and with the help of the oxygen, I was breathing better.

The Dr. was still refusing to give Hydrocortisone but wanted to do an x-ray and CT of my chest to see if there might be a tear in my lungs or a blood clot. I told him it was part of Addisons, and he said, "No. Those are not symptoms of an adrenal crisis symptoms." He said since my BP was "normal" (My normal BP is about 118/50 give or take – He thinks that 111/75 is normal). I get that with Addison's, BP tends to be very low, but I was also hyperventilating, so of course it was going to be high.

All the tests (for a heart attack) came back normal... I was discharged and now I am at home resting... and pissed.

This should not be happening to us. We need to raise awareness and be heard. Too many of our Addisonian friends are dying because Drs. are too arrogant and ignorant to listen to their patients. We have a voice and we need it to be heard.

I was lucky that I stress dosed that morning, right before I went to the ER, and when I was there, and they weren't in the room.

July 6, 2018

Today I felt a lot better. Got about 7 hours of sleep last night (didn't get out of bed til 11am). I was able to walk. I jumped on Instagram and called out some celebrities that I felt might be into stepping up and helping to raise some awareness for Addisons. I am tired of not being heard in the medical setting. They should know about this disease. I get that it is a rare disease, but I feel that if the ER department is brought in a patient who has a rare disease, the ER department should look into and educate their providers about it. It doesn't seem like it would be that hard to do.

Every time I have to stress dose, I get a bladder infection. It drives me nuts. Like my body doesn't already do enough weird shit, now I have to deal with painful urination.

On a good note, I am able to eat without pain and nausea, and just a little bit of bloating, so the Exlax/water thing worked. It also could have been what sent me into a crisis, so… I wouldn't recommend doing that unless your doctor approves…. which they might not.

July 11, 2018

Yesterday was another "exciting" day. I woke up feeling weak. Again, feeling like I had run a marathon. Every time I did anything, I was trying to catch my breath, even just talking. My youngest had an appointment with our naturopath, and so I asked if I could be seen at the same time. All morning I was just weak. I had to cancel my therapy appointment because I couldn't get out of bed.

When we got to the naturopath, I felt really dizzy getting out the car. My youngest helped me walk in. The receptionist said that I looked like I was having a rough day. We went back to the room and waited for a bit. I had to use the bathroom, so I got up and the room started to spin, I barely made it to the door and grabbed onto the display cabinet and then my naturopath caught me before I hit the floor. I was so dizzy. My BP was 80/46. Finally made it to the bathroom and back to the room, with lots of help walking from my naturopath.

We went over my son's blood work (since he was the reason we were there), and it turns out that he is very anemic, low DHEA, and his little adrenals are trying to work hard to keep up. As we were going through all of this, they hooked me up to a saline bag, to help my body out. With the dizziness and shortness of breath, that was getting worse, she wanted me to go to the ER, just to make sure everything was fine.

On the way to the ER, my breathing, or lack thereof, was getting worse. My friend who was taking me, was scared I was going to pass out. She said a couple times, there was a break in my breathing, and she had to look over to see if I was still with her.

The ER, again, didn't really help. I got my breathing under control and that was about it. The Dr. said that they can only treat what I came in for, which makes sense, but that I really need to be on top of all my symptoms and letting all my specialists know, because something is causing these breathing episodes.

The only thing that has changed in the last couple weeks is the fact that I started doing the meal replacement/protein shakes. My naturopath thinks it's a good idea to stop doing them for a while to see if these symptoms go away.

I also haven't pooped since early am on the 7th. I will be stopping the shakes, making my own electrolyte drink, and seeing how that goes. Here's hoping.

July 13, 2018

The past couple days have been good. After I stopped taking the meal replacement/protein shakes, my body has been doing better. I started making my own electrolyte drink, since my body has a hard time hanging onto hydration. I don't understand why, but I am doing everything I can to make it function better.

Found out on that my youngest is really anemic, low DHEA, and his little adrenals are having to work a little harder. So I got him on some iron, DHEA, and adrenal support vitamins, plus some vitamin D, because we live in Western Washington and we need it.

I haven't been sleeping good, which is not unusual, but I really want some good sleep.

I've been trying to keep up my activity by going to the gym. Sometimes I am embarrassed by my little tiny workouts, but I also don't want to overdo it.

My middle son got a job, and still hasn't told me about it. He found out 3 days ago. I don't know why he hasn't said anything to me. Makes me sad that he doesn't want to share that exciting news with me.

Trying to eliminate stress from my life, but how do you do that? I can't keep focusing on all the negative. Gotta try to stay positive.

July 14, 2018

The last couple days have been pretty good. Sleep is shitty as usual, but I do feel like I have some energy. I have been drinking 30oz of my homemade electrolyte drink along with 4 water bottles (40oz each) a day. I have been making sure I am eating (avoiding the shakes) at least 3 meals a day, and if I can fit in a snack, that's great.

10 days til I see the gastroenterologist. I am still getting the bloating, but it's not as severe, and still have a little bit of nausea. I am just thankful the horrible stomach pain stopped.

If it was the shakes that were making me have the breathing issues, I wonder what it is in them that caused that?

July 17, 2018

I have had a good few days. Exhaustion is the only thing I have been really dealing with. Which I can handle. There has still been some bloating and nausea with eating, but hopefully that will all be figured out soon. My oldest son and I leave today for his WSU orientation. I am excited to be able to get to spend some mom/son time with him before he goes off to college. I am glad that we get to go to the orientation together. This will help give me some peace of mind while he is there.

I have been drinking my electrolyte drink and I think that has been helping. Not that I have had a ton of energy, but I do feel better in a sense.

I got a letter from Disability and I have a court date set. Finally! It will be at the end of September, so I am going to have to make sure they get all the documentation and letters from my Drs. I really hope this goes in my favor. It has been such a fight. I am not doing this with a Lawyer, but I hope that I can win still.

July 19, 2018

Day 2 at orientation and my body is so pissed at me. I slept for about 3 hours and I know it was really shitty sleep. I was up at 5:30am and knew that it was going to be a long day…. and lots of walking.

Yesterday was so hard. Everything is up hill. They are not joking when they say "cougar calves." My body was already sore from all the walking up hills and around campus.

Today there was a lot more sitting, but still a shit ton of walking. College information overload. I took so many notes. When the first session was over, I got up to use the bathroom. I was extremely dizzy and nauseous. I am still having issues with eating, so it has not been good. I was glad that I would only be walking down stairs for the next session. After that I started to feel better. My body was screaming though.

The heat played a big part in how I was feeling as well. It was so hot, lots of walking (uphill), the going into an air conditioned building, walking some more… Repeat.

This experience was amazing and I am so glad that I got to come and experience it with him. I do have to say though, it was a lot for my body. I ended up having to miss 2 of the last sessions because I had to rest. I was in too much pain to try and keep going. I was trying to pace myself, but I also wanted to get in every session I possibly could. I just over did it, but it's done. I didn't participate in any of the night activities, because my body will not allow it. Would I have liked to? Yes. They had some really cool things going on for the students and parents. I am glad my son went out and enjoyed himself.

I was looking at all these other parents, and I don't know most of their stories, but I could tell the ones who could withstand the orientation festivities, and I envy them. I wish I could do all the things my body wants. I shouldn't complain, because I can still do a lot, but then I look back on what I used to do, and this is nothing compared to that.

July 21, 2018

After these long couple days of walking up 5 million hills, my body was in so much pain and so sore (some of it the good workout sore). I was so happy to go to sleep in my own bed.

I slept pretty good last night. I fell asleep really fast (around midnight) and didn't wake up til 10:45am. I did toss and turn a lot, but I got about 7 hours of motionless sleep (according to my tracker).

When I got up, I did feel like I needed to go back to sleep, but I had so much to get caught up gone since I was gone for a few days. I still feel really tired, so I am hoping that I will be able to get good sleep tonight.

I will say that I woke up with about a level 3 pain. I was really surprised that I wasn't in more pain, so I was really happy with that, but the fatigue is slowing me down.

July 24, 2018

Yesterday I felt a little bit normal from the WSU trip. We also decided to get the house moved around a bit. I knew that it would be a lot on my body doing it but didn't realize how hard. I woke up so sore. My husband stayed home from work and helped me move everything around, but it was still a lot.

I felt like the Princess and the Pea last night sleeping on my bed. I took off one of the mattress pads, and it didn't fair well for me. Hoping tonight (put the other pad back on) I will be able to get better sleep. I won't be so sore and stressed out from moving things around as well.

Was supposed to see the gastroenterologist today, but she was sick and had to reschedule. I am seeing her on Thursday. My first thought was, is she still going to be sick when she sees me? Will she pass her sickness on to me? I know that is not what I am supposed to be worried about, but having Addison's and a shitty immune, I can't risk it. I just need to invest in one of those masks that keep the germs away. I know they have really cool ones with awesome designs.

Trying to figure out my emotions. I am so all over the place with having to go see the new Drs. I want answers and they just seem out of reach at the moment.

July 25, 2018

Today has been so rough. I am so glad that it just happened to be a day that I had nothing going on. I stayed in bed til about 12:30pm. Laid around all day. Not by choice, my body just didn't have any energy to do anything.

I really wanted to do things today. I wanted to go to the gym, I wanted to clean out the car, I wanted to take my youngest to the lake…. but I just couldn't do it.

Every time I get up, I feel dizzy and got hit with a wave of exhaustion. I feel like I have to close my eyes and just sleep. These days are the hardest because I just don't know how to handle it mentally. It's a fight…. all the time…. I just hate this so much.

Depression really hits the hardest on these days. My inner voice is telling me how worthless I am and that my family deserves better than this. I know it's wrong, but it is really loud and convincing on these days.

Today the depression was at a high. I was feeling worthless and hopeless, like I don't have a place at all. I was defeated and beaten down.

My oldest son called me. He was needing me. He needed his mom. I know that I was there for him in his time of need, but he was the one who was there for me. We talked through what he was going through until he was done and then we said our goodbyes. He doesn't know it, but he lifted me up higher than I have been in a long time. He didn't know how important that phone call was to me, he just knew that I was there for him when he needed me, and as a mom, that felt amazing.

July 26, 2018

Today I went to see the gastroenterologist. I was pleasantly surprised at her knowledge and excitement about Addisons Disease. She seemed pretty thrilled to have a patient with it since it's so rare, but that just made me feel good about her. She answered all my questions and also was able to make the connection of my symptoms to having Addisons on top of the other issues. She told me something I didn't even realize and that was that with having Addisons disease, my body will have a harder time staying hydrated, so I need to try extra hard to get in the electrolytes to keep me where I need to be. She wants to do a gallbladder ultrasound since that is where my stomach seems to be the most sensitive to pressure. Then at the end of August I have a endoscopy and colonoscopy scheduled on the same day. I am not to sure about that, but I guess the good thing is, is I will get a good pipe cleaning. Fun times!!

Today was a lot better than yesterday. I am having trouble with the heat this year. I have swelling and daily headaches. I get way too hot and feel like I can't function. This has not been an issue in the past. Heat has always been my friend and now I am struggling with it.

I have been extremely tired all day and I think that has to do with having to be up so early for my appointment.

I am glad I was pulled out of my funk a bit today. I don't think I could have handled a "depression" day like yesterday again. I was able to get up and meal prep some pasta salads, because it's been too hot to use the oven.

Last night a mosquito decided to violate my body 8 times. I have so many bites and I was itchy all night. 5 bites on my hand, 1 on my shoulder, 1 on my forearm, and 1 on my leg. Little bastard. I hope he died from all that blood. Tonight, I need the sleep, so I am hitting the hay early.

July 30, 2018

Today was a little better than the past few days. I was able to make it to the gym. Thank God that the YMCA has a kid swim thing that my youngest loves to go to. That way, I can workout while he has fun swimming with other kids for a couple hours. I really needed to get out of the house.

I did a lot of laying around on the weekend, watching Parenthood, and just feeling depressed. Went for a walk on Sunday to try and pull myself out of the depression, but that didn't work so well. It was painful on my back to walk. The weather was great, but the pain was just a bit too much. Spent the rest of the day on the couch.

So glad I had therapy today. I really needed to talk through some things. With the upcoming school year, I want to be prepared a LOT more than I was the previous year. My youngest really threw me for a loop and I realized just how unprepared I was for it. I don't want it to be a fail, so I am really going to cater it to his liking so it's not so overwhelming and hopefully he will enjoy learning and not make it so difficult.

I am also wanting to set up a better schedule for me to follow so I am not overwhelmed.

I got a new shake to try. This one only has 5 ingredients, so hopefully I won't have to go to the ER again. I really like how this one tastes.

I am anxious about getting the colonoscopy and endoscopy. I don't want them done, but I know they are necessary. It seems that every 2 years, something autoimmune comes into play, so I hope that is not the case. I just hope everything comes back fine and the symptoms all go away, and I can live a normal, happy life. I know, stupid, but that is what I am hoping for.

July 31, 2018

Went to see the new neurologist today. She was a little different. She didn't seem very social and kind of seemed like she didn't even want to be there. When she brought up how depressed I was, she seemed irritated that I am choosing not to be medicated for it, or like she didn't believe that I wasn't suicidal. I can't really say that I didn't or did like her, but I will be seeing her again mid-September. She is sending me in for a brain MRI, so that will be set up soon. She was very thorough with the tests she did in the office. My other neurologist never did any of that stuff. I can deal with a stand-offish Dr., because that is definitely better than a prideful one who won't listen to you.

I got a call from the gastroenterologist and my gallbladder ultrasound came back looking great, so that is a plus. I didn't think there would be anything wrong with my gallbladder, but apparently, she had the concern…. or just wanted to make me pay more…

Went to see my surgeon today too. He doesn't know why my back is still bothering me. He wants to do a CT scan to see if the bone actually healed the way it was supposed to. We are thinking that maybe because of the Addison's and having to take steroids that the bone didn't heal like we hoped or maybe even not at all. If that is the case, then we will know what to do when the scans come back. With all these scans I am getting and exposure to radiation, I hope that I get some super power…. like the ability to heal myself. Wouldn't that be so cool?!?! I watch way too many movies.

My last outing for the day was the massage appointment. I wish I had a really good therapist who could do all the things my body needed. I will be on the hunt for one soon, since this is my last appointment with this lady. The plus side is, she is from Dublin, so I get to listen to her accent.

Tonight, after I ate I had horrible bloating. It was extremely painful. I am so tired of this and wish that my endoscopy/colonoscopy would have been scheduled earlier. It's not fun dealing with this pain and I think that it should be taken more seriously and not scheduled out a month. When people can't eat because of pain, I think that constitutes as somewhat of an emergency and that they should be seen sooner than a month. I feel like I am being a baby about it, but then again, I also have the right to complain because it is true. How many people need this procedure done on a daily basis that they are so booked, that it takes a month to get in, yet I can get in for an MRI in about 2 days?? That just doesn't make any sense.

I will just sleep today off. It was a lot on my body and I am ready for bed.

******

Here it is, the beginning of all new tests and awaiting results. This is the worst part for me, the not knowing what to expect (if anything). Drs. schedule things so far out that it makes me so crazy and anxious.

I hope that I will not end up with anything new, but there are lots of tests and scans I still have to go through and then I will get some answers. Until then, it is just the stressful waiting game.

I will continue to pray that everything is ok. I will continue my vegan diet and I will continue to exercise when my body allows it. I can't stop my life, I am already super depressed, so I will keep myself busy.

The results will come when they come. When I get some answers, I will continue to write about the findings, my health, and my story. Thank you for reading and I hope this has helped you in some way. I look forward to sharing more of my life with you all.

SICK MOM CONFESSION

I feel like I have lost everything I am, not that I really knew who I was to begin with. Being a young mom, that is all I have ever really been; always taking care of others. Now that I am sick, it's hard to let others take care of me. After going hard for over 30 years, it's not easy to just give up that power.

Being a sick mom isn't easy. I don't like my kids seeing my bad days, and I really don't want them too have to take care of me or miss out on things because I can't go. I know that they want the best for me and they don't care that I have to miss out on some of their activities, but I feel like a horrible mom and they don't see it that way at all.

I miss being their healthy mom. I miss the activities and the energy that kept me going. I think about all the things we could be doing as a family if I didn't have these limitations. I think about the memories we could be making. I just need to stop, because that shit is depressing. I can still make memories, they might not be as good, but it's still time with them, no matter what we are doing. They will remember that; I need to remember that it's good enough for them. Being with me is enough for them and feeling loved by me is enough for them.

We can easily go into a depression and let these diseases consume us. We can dwell on the what if's all day. But that takes away from the memories we could be making. It takes away a little bit of our sanity. It's not easy. It's fucking hard to let it go. I have been dealing with this for almost 4 years…. That's nothing. I have been dealing with lower back pain for over 8 years now. I am still here. I am still alive. I can still have a life that I can be proud of. I can still watch my boys achieve everything they set out to do. That to me is something worth fighting for.

This is a war. Daily casualties are expected. They can be as minor as showers, getting dressed or as big as losing jobs and relationships. Each casualty hurts no matter how big or small. It's a part of you that you lose. The war is lost but there are still battles going on, so you have to keep fighting those. The small wins give us hope for the next battle. Don't be afraid to call in recruitments; friends, family, and even strangers. Let them help you win these battles.

We need to learn to triage. What can wait and what needs to be dealt with now. Learn to be ok with letting the little things go. Things can wait til you are feeling better. Not everything has to be done now. Not everything is an emergency. I am the worst at this, because I want it all done right now. Still learning how to triage myself, so be patient with yourselves.

Looking back at the stresses I dealt with as a healthy mom vs the stresses I have to deal with as a sick mom, I've felt the effects on me in both situations. Now it's way more painful and can take me out for a few days or send me into a crisis, but the hurt was still there when I was healthy, just in a different way. I was just better equipped to make it through it...a glass of wine helped too.

I have SO MUCH guilt from being sick; it's frustrating. It's how I see me, not how others see me. It's the failure I think I am, yet my kids, husband, and friends only see the fight in me. They see how brave I pretend to be and the struggle I go through. They want to help and encourage me, but I get so caught up in my guilt that I can't see my own positive impact.

I am a huge believer in "things happen for a reason." I would like too know why God chose me to handle this life I now have to live, but I know that he has a good reason. Even though I might not see it yet, it's there. Whether it benefits me or benefits you, or my boys, or someone out there. It is His reason and I am ok with that. I will live my life the best I can. I will share my story and hope it inspires others. I will step up and raise awareness. I will enjoy the time that I have with my boys, fighting every day; because they are my strength. I need to let their positive voices outshine my inner negative voice.

I hope you can find your strength. Keep fighting every day! You are badass....

ABOUT THE AUTHOR

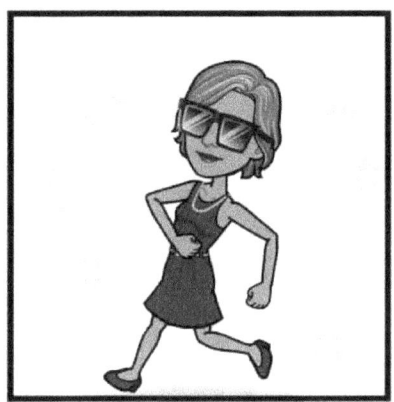

Let me start by introducing myself. I am a fiery mix of bitch and sarcasm with a hint of sweetness... or maybe that's just the perfume of those woman who pass me by. I am a mother of 3 boys!! Yes, I got lucky, I get the joys of being a boymom. I love every burp, fart, nose pick, and pee all over the toilet.

I LOVE running, like LOVE LOVE running. It's such an amazing stress reliever and it's the reason I haven't killed anyone yet. I love working out in general and hot yoga. Nothing like sweating with a bunch of strangers (unless you have to fart).

So here I am today, my body fucking hates me and tries to kill me off daily. I had to quit the job I loved and was amazing at (yes, I was amazing, you can ask my clients). Had to stop running because my chronic back pain and 2 surgeries haven't been any help. But now I get to write about it and hopefully raise some much needed awareness. I will keep it real; no sugar coating here. Enjoy the blunt, uncut shit I call life. Laugh, cry, drink, smoke; do what you need to, as you enter my life.

Follow me on social media to keep up with my crazy life:
Instagram: @chronic_moms_club
Blog: chronicmomsclub.wixsite.com/chronicmomsclub
Email: chronicmomsclub@gmail.com